NEEDWOOD

A year in search of ordinary things.

MILES RICHARDSON

Published in 2012 by FeedARead.com Publishing – Arts
Council funded
Copyright © Miles Richardson.

A CIP catalogue record for this title is available from the
British Library.

THE LANDSCAPE AROUND NEEDWOOD

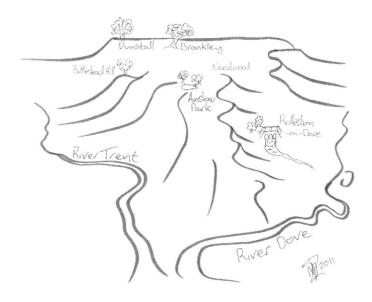

CONTENTS

Introduction   My Natural Health Service

I   Detail of Winter

II   Finding Nature

III   Hawks

IV   Connected

V   Spanish Plume

VI   Soundscapes of the Dales

VII   Equinox

VIII   The Darkness of Midsummer

IX   Extraordinary Things

X   The Dove

XI   The Stealing

XII   The Closing

INTRODUCTION

MY NATURAL HEALTH SERVICE

Many of us are intuitively aware of the benefits of spending time in the natural world and my natural health service lies on the higher ground between two wide alluvial valleys, home to the River Dove to the north and the River Trent to the east. This land was once home to the wild and ancient Needwood Forest, granted by Henry III to his son Edmund in 1267 and thereby into the possession of the Duchy of Lancaster: over 9400 acres of wood pasture used for hunting by kings and divided into wards and great estates that have now faded. The forest trees were mostly oak, lime, hazel, maple and hawthorn, with few beech or elm. When parliament passed legislation to divide, allot and enclose it in the early 1800s, a long period of deforestation began. Eventually, all but 500 acres of the forest were removed, leaving just a few dozen veteran oaks, up to 700 years old, in some of the country's most ancient oak woodland in the areas that were difficult to farm. The area is now mainly agricultural, presenting a rural English landscape of rolling hills, rich pastoral land, Enclosure Act hedgerows, ash and oaks.

The Dove has a catchment in the wetter uplands of the Peak District, and often the river breaks free from its banks onto the level fields of the flood plain. These flat water meadows and pasture provide a great expanse, backed by trees and grazed by cattle. Close to where the Dove meets the Trent the principal town clings to the river and spreads out onto the flood plain.

In many ways this is an ordinary English landscape. This simplicity is its appeal, but also a limitation. There is no obvious grandeur, wilderness or drama. So I seek out and enjoy the ordinary things: the oak, the rook, the sky. The solace of the risings, the calm of the water meadows and the lifeless hedgerows of winter under a leaden sky.

Of course, I'm not the first to find calm in nature. Back in 1801 the romantic poet Samuel Taylor Coleridge wrote of the soothing effect of nature. But nature is not just soothing; it can have real health benefits. In his 1836 essay *Nature*, Ralph Waldo Emerson noted how nature restores mind and body from the effects of harmful work. With an attentive eye, Emerson found delight in the "glory and gloom" of winter scenery and the simple changes in the natural landscape that occur and are gone in each passing moment.

This realisation of the benefits of, and need for, interaction with the natural landscape was also expressed in 1854 by Henry Thoreau when he wrote about simple living in natural surroundings in his book *Walden*. He understood the link between well-being and nature and the interaction between our internal world and the external environment:

"There can be no very black melancholy to him who lives in the midst of nature and has his senses still."

To go right back, Hippocrates made the link between the environment and health over 2000 years ago in *Airs, Waters and Places*. This is all very good, but I am also interested in understanding why there is a link and what happens in our minds when we experience nature. In 1865 the landscape architect Frederick Law Olmsted showed a particularly insightful understanding of this relationship and gave reasons why the contemplation of natural scenes is favourable for mental and physical health. He wrote of attention being aroused and the mind being occupied without purpose, which is in line with some of today's thinking as to why natural environments are good for health and well-being. A common theme amongst several of these theories is that people benefit from interactions with the environment in which they evolved, the environment for which they are innately adapted. As this evolution took place over millions of years, and urbanisation is in comparison a recent blink, it would seem to be a sensible idea. Humans may well be adaptable, but we can't just discard our pre-history; perhaps that's why many of us enjoy having a living flame in our living rooms.

Thankfully, it seems that a restorative cure for urban living is to put on our boots and get out into the landscape. We are hard-wired to find the natural world calming and the everyday stress that threatens our well-being can be reduced by viewing the landscape. This allows the eyes to extend their visual field and take in the subtle complexity of the natural surroundings that capture our attention, restrict intrusive thoughts and allow tension, heart rate and blood pressure to return to lower levels. Nature is not just about restoration, though. Nature can boost our vitality, help us flourish and function well, both personally and socially.

Clearly something interesting happens in our minds when we go out into the natural world, and I believe knowing a little about this can enhance our enjoyment. So, before my year-long search begins and we enter the external natural world, let us journey a little way into our internal world. For example, here's something that amazes me: whatever we experience in the world, what we see, hear and feel, meaning is derived from the things we perceive and the memories they evoke. If you think about this, it means that no two people ever experience the same scene in precisely the same way. When we stand with others looking out over the landscape we each take something different from the same view.

This evaluation of the things our senses bring into our minds – that is, assigning value and experiencing feeling or emotion – is termed "affect". This is a top-down process driven from within our internal world and therefore reflects our personality, attitudes and beliefs, which is why some of us might feel the need to run away if we saw a snake during our natural wanderings, or not go out in the first place.

Affect is important. It is the constant companion of sensation and we have an affective system that controls our muscles and the way our brain functions. Positive affect, which is boosted by immersion in and connectedness to nature, is relaxing; chemicals flood through the brain, broadening our processing and horizons. With negative affect we focus on an issue, and our muscles tense, ready to respond: very useful to our ancestors when they were threatened by a nasty snake, but frustrating to us when we ruminate on a deadline at work or someone's unkindness.

Our complex brains go beyond these automatic and rapid visceral level responses. A behavioural level controls our actions and influences our base visceral processing. Finally, a reflective level allows us to consciously reflect on experiences and this biases behaviour. At the visceral level we respond positively to things the natural world provides, such as climate, colour, melody, symmetry, smooth shapes and sounds, although we are all different and have acquired tastes driven by our reflective mind. At the base level, humans must have always found pleasure in the natural world through our senses; the warmth of the sun or a cooling breeze. Our ability to reflect and think has also seen pleasure through creativity, such as producing cave paintings of the wild animals around us.

This simple description of our brain suggests that the reflective, behavioural and visceral responses reflect its evolution, back through time from reflective human, to behavioural mammals, to visceral reptiles simply responding to threats and opportunities. This evolution, rather than design, is a possible reason for some human ailments, with an imbalance between the three being seen as a cause of conditions such as depression where our threat response is overactive and our positive affect is reduced. To feel good we need emotional balance; happiness and contentment comes through balancing threat, desire and affiliation.

We've almost wandered into the territory of self-help, but help from what? Well, earlier I mentioned urban living and that Emerson noted the ill effects of noxious work. So why did our ancestors ever leave nature behind? We can blame technology and our innate design skills driven by our imaginative human mind – our technology shapes and defines us more and more. Technological advances first allowed people to settle, to farm the land, but further advances eventually saw people leave the fields and villages for an industrial, contrasting life in towns and cities where, now, many of us live in debt-funded and closely packed dwellings. We are trapped into this lifestyle, where work is no longer driven by the seasons and we are detached from the environment of our evolution. We now enjoy the natural world as observers, on the outside, detached from it in the Anthropocene age. We are products of nature trapped inside human beings, trapped by our technology; the technology we would now struggle to survive without. We are of nature, but not in it.

Whilst our modern life is preferable to that of our predecessors in many ways, our consumerist society has created new pressures. Sometimes we need to walk away from these pressures and as we have seen, the natural environment is a good place to do this. A gentle and effortless connectedness to nature helps give meaningful purpose to our lives, improves well-being and allows reflection.

Establishing this connection can be facilitated by taking time to appreciate ordinary things and to engage more fully with nature. Life is now rapid and we rarely pause to appreciate the moment. This, together with the soft fascination of nature, allows an uncomplicated state of mind similar to mindfulness, directing attention without evaluation to the present moment – doing less and noticing more. Nan Shepherd captured this well in *The Living Mountain* when she wrote of the landscape giving most when she had no destination.

Adopting a mindful approach enhances the sensory impact of nature and can strengthen our connectedness to the natural world. However, like sleep, it cannot be forced, but we have to make it possible and the natural environment is an ideal place to do this. Simply paying attention and being more aware of the details around us and the thoughts and feelings they produce. This gives the mind a chance to settle and experience itself differently as we become increasingly conscious of being conscious. This highlights the key difference between the nature we observe and us; we know we are alive. The life around us lives and dies not knowing that it exists, which makes me wonder how can we have destroyed so much of nature, when it is only beautiful to our eyes?

We have seen that our need for, and experience of nature is tied to the interface between the internal and external world, and this interface between the external natural world and internal mind is the focus of this book. Not a dry scientific account, but the simple notes of my interaction with the landscape, the stimuli within it and my response. The sights, sounds and sensations that enter my mind and where they take me as I search for ordinary natural things over the course of a year. This brings us to the following notes from my ramblings in the landscape and my journey from attentiveness and observation to connection as the landscape flows into my mind and I hear nature's voice.

I

DETAIL OF WINTER

3 January to 23 February

After a day beneath a static blanket of blue grey cloud, brightness came and there was time to begin my search for ordinary things. At Anslow Park the sun, our ordinary star, was low in the sky and intense in the reflection from the pond that had been frozen for a few weeks. It extracted and teased the remnants of colour from the reeds and I could see little more than the light and shade of the mounds of grass on the path before me. Attentive, I sensed the faint breath of cold air flowing through the hedgerows, occasional birdsong could be heard, a lone rabbit ran into the field and two blackbirds passed through the young trees in front of me. On rising to the highest ground I looked out across the Trent Valley. To the west of the monumental cooling towers that stand proud at Willington, I could see the cream spillage of the car factory lying across the landscape; the landscape to be searched for ordinary natural things.

Winter days can have seemingly little to offer and a few days later, with the thaw complete, the cold was from the biting wind. With the previous day's snow gone and the ground no longer frozen it was sodden underfoot and I watched the water covering the top of my boots with each mindful step. The pond at Anslow Park was considerably deeper, with water audibly flowing in from the fields above. The sky had been clear, but there was only the occasional shaft of sunlight and for a short time it was directed at me, reflecting brightly off the wet leaves fallen from the oak, which became silver stepping-stones to higher ground. I looked out again, north across the Dove Valley towards the

1

Peak District, to the faint signs of snow on the tops around Ashbourne and Matlock. To the south a thick grey blanket of cloud sat above a rim of pale peach brightness on the horizon.

Returning to Rolleston in more reliable late afternoon sun, I hoped to see the kingfisher. I feel that I have to believe it will appear, but not expect to see it. I stood by the Alderbrook enjoying the silence. I must have been over-confident as there was little more to see than the solid brown water in the swollen brook. I returned via the woods of Brook Hollows with the low sun turning orange behind the trees. A wren popped by and closer to home a large flock of pigeons passed overhead with a crescent moon behind them. There was detail, but scant connection.

A brisk wind breathed life into the hedgerows of January. The trees stood ready for the action of spring and the holly brought a few red spots of colour. To the north, west and south there was a thick bank of cloud, but it was clearer to the east, but no chance of sun, just a few splashes of rain as I walked beneath a tree brought to life by a hundred starlings chattering and a lone pigeon providing the bass line – hardly Bootsy Collins, but a real ordinary pleasure.

Later in the day, walking through a ribbon of pine trees at Blithfield, there seemed little to observe, just the bright green moss attempting to climb the tree trunks. I left the wood to cross the meadow, now bare and stony, yet full of red poppies last summer. Over the stile a fallen branch lay helpless, covered in lime- and olive-coloured lichens, with leaf-buds formed and ready. The path drops and winds through this deciduous wood and it was peaceful. It was good to stop and be surrounded, to try and sense connection. An ancient oak stripped of bark stood with me, looking out over the dark pool where several tree stumps protruded through the surface. The path had a natural carpet of oak leaves, their autumn colours drained, apart from those that lay in the shallows of the pool, which reflected some welcome colour to my eyes. On the shores of the reservoir the uninterrupted wind whipped freely. Four ducks emerged keenly and headed into the wind only to drop to the water moments later. A sole gull passed overhead. An uprooted beech lay beneath another, with its multitude of fine branches reaching upward from a squat trunk. It offered husks to me as I passed, but I hadn't discovered how to receive them. The wind dropped and the lapping water could be heard. Further on, in a calmer stretch, the still water reflected the light to create a ribbon of white, when suddenly the sun broke through and the drab landscape was brought to life for an instant, lifted by a yellow hue, and then was gone. An ordinary, but magical, end.

To deal with my new attentiveness to the external world, my mind must form new internal connections that take time and continued engagement. So the next day I continued to accept the detail of winter and I watched closely as a single oak leaf spun and tumbled down slowly, as if it was trying to avoid landing on the lake, which still had a large expanse of ice in a shaded bay. Just above the trees a brilliantly bright ball of blue grey cloud gave away the position of the sun. The cloud thinned enough on occasion to allow the light to flow forth, picking out the birches on the water's edge opposite. A single bulrush pointed to the sky. A few steps further and yet more white birch stood on a small headland, their reflections in the water creating the image of mammoth jaws waiting to pounce. For somewhere so modest I find this old gravel pit quite enchanting, especially the natural lawns of grass in the clearings surrounded by the birch. Further on, the stumps of a dozen or so birch stood a few feet high, guarding a pool whilst their tall slender brothers and sisters stood behind them swaying in the wind, perhaps twenty metres high. My young children, Leon and Isla, played below, digging out rotten tree stumps with sticks, finding glistening yellow spheres that looked like slugs' eggs to my

3

untrained eye. Whilst waiting, I wandered over a small embankment and found a horned black sheep with a rather menacing stare. As we set off back there was just enough sunlight to cast a shadow and it gave a crisp white highlight to the edge of each birch trunk.

After seven hours confined, the fresh air felt especially crisp. There was an enveloping grey-orange confusion of fuzzy clouds and a few drops of rain. Given my confinement I would have been content with a functional three-mile stroll, but as I crossed the Alderbrook at the ford there it was, the kingfisher perched on a tree twenty yards away. A hot glowing coal, apparent in the fading light. It allowed me a few seconds and then it was off and away a few feet above the water. I set off again with, it is true to say, a spring in my step, only to find yet more pleasure. The confusion of clouds had formed into fine sunset, grey purple clouds backlit to produce an outline of gold, and the clouds to the side had their shape picked out in an almost pink hue. And above a strip of milky blue sky with the odd grey smudge of a shower was a dark mass of cloud with an underbody of orange, like the robin behind me, which was providing the soundtrack to my viewing.

The dark evenings limited time and it was a week before I was able to continue my search. It was a still and frosty day, with the air too dry to ice glass. I set off in search of a tree that had stood out to me for thirty years. As a child looking out from our front room it had stood slender and silhouetted against the setting sun. Although a little ungainly, it has always had a certain simple elegance, tall with a long trunk and a couple of branches up top that support a sparse lopsided oval of foliage in the summer. Over the past few weeks I had triangulated its position from viewpoints on a few of my regular walks. When checking the map it revealed it was close to a lane I wasn't aware of. I found it to be a cold and exposed spot within a couple of hundred yards of my target, but I couldn't identify the exact position on the map. I decided to try to approach the tree via a footpath from the opposite side. Again I got within a couple of hundred yards and, looking up at the tree, was able to locate its position relative to the field boundaries with more accuracy: 52°50'07.6"N, 1°40'01.2"W. On my way back around the edge of a few recently ploughed fields I found a dead buzzard lying on its back, its breast feathers unkempt, yellow feet clenched, claws rendered pathetic, and haunting opaque grey eyes robbed of their fire. From its size I felt it might have hatched last year. I walked on next to the Alderbrook towards the hollows. There had been no hint of sunshine, but suddenly the fields were lit. I was in the shadow of the trees, but soon emerged into glorious, truly golden light. I felt so tall as my shadow stretched out before me, a perfect chill on my face; it was a visceral and reflective moment. My mind was as clear as the air and I was content. I stood and soaked up the light and became aware of all the sounds around me. General chattering, rustling and the whirring beat of a pigeon's wings as it ventured through the trees. This was a memorable moment. It felt like a moment of connection. An alarm-like call attracted my attention. It was a nuthatch, and I watched as it went on a gravity-defying walk underneath the branches.

Another week passed and into February. A heavy day, dense cloud and strong winds. In Brook Hollows, Leon and Isla paddled, unblocking the stream underneath the bridge so that the clear water could flow. I stood and could feel the raindrops on my skin, hear the faint tap as they hit my hat and see the snowdrops quiver in the wind. Truly sensational.

My attention turned to the waterfall. Sheets of water breaking up into torrents and a white cascade on the rocks below. The ripples breaking up the light and dark as they approached me, nature flowing from the external to the internal. I watched a party of long-tailed tits skit, float and pause in the branches above.

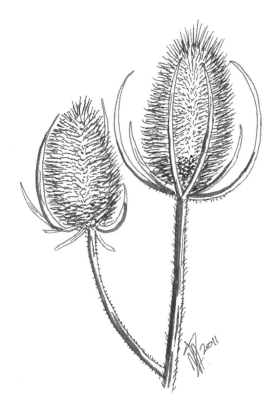

The following day at Anslow Park there was a relentless wind as I pushed on past the full pond, with choppy surface and reeds bent over. I sat here on a summer evening last year watching swifts and swallows skim the water. This time small birds were performing their own acrobatics as they fought the wind. The cloud hung low, deep and grey. Where there had been frost and reflected light, now there was mud and faded grass. On the hilltop, the large corner oak stood stubborn, with jaunty hazel catkins waving below. Nearby the silver-grey furry catkins of a willow and teasels stood together, at opposite ends of the tactile spectrum, creating a wild sensory garden. Beneath the bands of grey and white cloud fading into the horizon the winter countryside was laid bare. Half a dozen finches appeared and did battle with the wind before falling to the ground. A wood pigeon powered past and the finches rose again, this time travelling with the wind.

I chose to stand by the ford in the Alderbrook for five minutes. A black cat and a blackbird were in the adjacent field. Then the cat was gone and there was a pair of blackbirds, tails cocked, chasing across the grass. They flew a few feet into a nearby bush. There was constant birdsong all around, pigeons, tits, robins and their like. A large fox casually crossed the open field and a single blackbird returned before shooting off with a call of alarm. I noticed the willow; suddenly a subtle cascade of lime green reflected in the brook, thousands of leaves encouraged to emerge. Mallards splashed and washed below as others approached, leaving a V-shaped wake in the still water behind. The crocuses were hot on the heels of the snowdrops and daffodils pointed skyward, ready to launch – commencing countdown, engines on.

At Dunstall we wandered along a track through one of the many newly planted woodlands in the area, and heard the characteristic high-pitched shriek of a buzzard flying ahead. The long needles of the Corsican pines glistened, several inches long in bushy throngs. Home for a ladybird, six black dots and one white, the sun reflected in the translucent orange shell. A lone crow sat on the uppermost branch of a tree nearby, surveying the field below, waiting for an opportunity as we rummaged amongst the pines. Then the crow swooped down through the trees, but only to an alternative perch. Leon found a more aggressive pine, with short jabbing needles. We moved on, by an old hedgerow towards an open field. Bright yellow cup lichens clung to a particular type of tree within the hedge, contrasting with the deep purple leaf-buds. Sheep had left narrow tracks radiating like veins across the field. Exploring the area for the first time, we had to force our way through a thorny hedge, going backwards, keeping close to avoid being struck as the spiked twigs flicked past. We took a detour past a rabbit burrow surrounded by fresh reddened soil as white cloud bubbled up to the west. A pair of buzzards swooped nearby, calling to each other as they went. We set off back, through established woodland once again, emerging at a high point where the fields fall away, steeply, but in a series of pleasing curves. Atop a skeletal ghost tree sat a buzzard, which then launched into flight. It joined another and they soared, their wings outstretched above our heads. The sun was low enough to light and reveal the underside of their wings. The occasional flick of their wing tips was sufficient to maintain the display for some time. The cloud became thick and grey, and rain threatened, but the sun hung on and, looking across to the hilltop, the shadows of several oak were cast down the hillside we had descended. Back home, the rain arrived, the sound pulsing with the gusts of the wind and then the song of a blackbird – what a voice!

The cold grey mass of the reservoir at Carsington was mirrored by the sky. We moved through a static landscape. Life was on hold, a pause button pressed until the relief of the constant twisting flow of a stream. Onwards and over the water a large flock of tufted ducks rose, twisted together for a little while and then returned to the surface. We walked on, in an environment that detached one from reality, with occasional birdsong like an alarm to awake me from a dream. A crow glided in to land as steady and controlled as an airliner on a final approach. And then another. As dusk took hold, the trees restricted to the hedgerows across the fields faded from clear view, flattened and black, fanning their intricate branches against a featureless grey backdrop until only the closest could be seen.

I was enjoying the detail in the landscape, extracting what I could from it, looking forward to a new day and a new experience in a familiar place. Lying beneath the sky, the waterlogged fields of Brankley gripped and pulled at my boots with every step. What had been a boggy ditch had become a fast-flowing stream. Brambles trailed into the water, resisting and disturbing the flow to create a restful babble. The rain was still falling, tapping out random rhythms. Furry catkins, decorated with water droplets, looked sugar-coated. I stood alone in the sodden landscape for some time to take it in. Raindrops hung like jewels from the buds on the otherwise bare birch, refracting all the light of the grey sky into a point of white, lifting the scene before me. In the wood, trails of water had marked out dark ribbons down the tree trunks. I emerged past ancient oak and holly into the pastureland where the most ancient oak had split since my last visit. A substantial branch torn from its host lay before me, revealing a hollow trunk. One main branch remained at one with the trunk. A pair of rabbits burst into view and bolted underneath the abandoned hut, which was surrounded by snowdrops and daffodils. I turned to take in the view across the fields below. A stream previously unknown to me had burst its banks and two cows stared at me, one black, one white, looking like primitive beasts as they stood motionless by a newly formed pool. I was stood beneath a snag tree with deep cracks running parallel along the trunk and onto the branches above. By the time I turned to return the rain band had passed and the teasels that had stood through the snow lay defeated. As the Earth turned away from the sun it seemed like every hundred yards there was the shrill call of another blackbird. They were in the hedgerows, on the field gates, in the trees and darting through the air. The water flowed, the Earth turned, the darkness spread over me and the birds still sang.

II

FINDING NATURE

24 February to 18 March

A day that felt like spring. The snowdrops and crocuses, yellow, lilac and white, were wide open, taking in the sun. But spring does not begin at a point in time, or space. Spring develops, driven by a climate change that occurs each year as the Earth travels around our star. Warmer days become more frequent, a trend tied to our orbit, to which the plants respond and the behaviour of the wildlife begins to change – just as behaviour changes each day as the Earth turns on its axis. The events that we perceive to signal spring have recently come earlier in our orbit, driven by our planet's climate changing. Forget the definitions: spring is a state of mind, it ebbs and flows, teases us and creeps upon us until a tipping point is reached. It becomes spring, a social construction.

My search for ordinary things continued with a first visit to Springwood, away from Needwood, near Calke Abbey on the border of Derbyshire and Leicestershire. The content was familiar. Established oak and then birch, bluebells in the green preparing for their show. Whilst exploring the new wood I disturbed a woodcock. It erupted from the woodland floor, angular head squat to body as it fled the scene.

I returned the next day to explore further as this place is quiet, undisturbed. Trees lay where they had fallen. A wren darted beneath us and a couple of great tits perched before us. We paused to watch a small bird silhouetted above us. It was nimble, hanging from catkins, a marsh tit, we decided. Then go-go-go, a crow cried directly above us as it forced a

11

buzzard away. Onward, a birch shorn of all branches stood, fungi clinging to its sides providing greasy footholds. We crept to the site of yesterday's woodcock, taking care of where we trod. There was nothing but a birch, lying on the shore as if drinking from the water. A great crested grebe swam by. A trio of cormorants, a pair of coots, the unsophisticated calls of waterbirds. The water lay flat, a bright mass balancing the sky, a ribbon of green between. The birch tightly packed, slender, swayed waiting for sunlight, leaves and energy. They were stark and honest, positive branches at acute angles reaching for the sky supporting a mass of wispy twigs. Nearby six or seven birch had fallen, or were well set to do so. Dozens of birch branches, recently felled, a tangle of twigs still attached, lay at the base of those remaining. A purple haze beneath columns of white on a canvas of copper ferns. A tawny owl called twice as the clouds allowed the sun to break through for the briefest moment. We descended through a clearing to the shore. It was cold as the tiny waves lapped at our feet. A pair of geese moaned as they went by. I turned as a single oak leaf fell, perceptually salient in the stillness as it descended alone to the grass, a reminder of autumn past. There were dark clouds behind; I thought the rain today had passed. It was a little too cold to hang around. I sought out some shelter from the wind as Leon patrolled the shoreline looking for a stick that wouldn't sink. Suddenly the sun made a transformational entrance. The water danced and the droplets on the birch highlighted the purple haze as tiny spits of rain fell in between to provide yet more lenses and mirrors to play with the light and kiss the sky. Then the scene became flat once again, the birch dense, the water grey, lifted only by the gentle lapping on the shore.

At home, the first daffodils had appeared and the rooks' nests were taking shape in the high branches. Yet it was a cold day with rain threatening as we set out, and Blithfield had few signs of spring. No snowdrops, no bluebells emerging and the pine trees had little change to offer. There was a cold wind and light rain. The pink and green buds of the hawthorn hedge drew my attention. The raindrops were crisp on the stiff leaves of the holly. A myriad of signals entered my mind which made sense of them, memories evoked and written in parallel. Young oaks stood waterlogged in the pools extended by the rain; the wind had dropped, the water was silent. It was calm. It was gentle. Like a still evening by the sea. I felt part of a contented world, not detached from it. The rain stopped. I heard a woodpecker's drum burst and general chatter from the woods behind. Things were picking up. The rain and wind returned, placing a mood-changing grey filter on my view. A lone goldfinch bounced by in front of three oaks with fractal snaking branches. The water surface fizzed with rain. And then it was still once more, apart from the rapid bidirectional ripples near the shore. A burst of sunlight swept over half the scene. It hung on, intense, reflected, warmth-giving. We stopped and the children played until circular ripples began to radiate on the water. Then it was churned into a pitted morass. A tractor towing rounded bales glided along the causeway in the distance, a dark grey silhouette against an olive grey skyline, topped and tailed by more grey tones. We were underneath our umbrellas, sheltered by the old fisherman's hut, which is black with a distinct whiff of creosote. The rain stopped again and we moved on. In the field, several grooves left by the wheels of a tractor were waterlogged and reflected the light as they converged into the distance.

With the sun falling, time was tight for my first outing of March. It was cloud-free except for a static patch of white painted on the milky blue, which faded to a yellow tinted white towards the low sun. The yellow light picked out the blades of grass in the fields and cast my shadow onto the hawthorn hedge and then thirty yards into the old orchard. The trees to the west were black, fading to grey. Layers of flat painted scenery faded to the horizon. To the east the trees had a faint glow. It was still and cold. The month had changed, an expectation of spring brought to mind, but the change is not dependent on the turning of a calendar. Three crows, then four, glistened amongst the lush grass as they fed. A robin, its red picked out by the sun, laid claim to its land through song from a perch high above. Birch and willow hung with grace, bright green or blackened against the light. The rooks were gathering, gliding, landing, but they couldn't settle. Two mallards flew west towards the horizon and my slender tree, which stood pink-grey through a barely detectable mist, the thin arc of the setting sun to one side. I felt a slow, but steady, understanding of the landscape developing.

At Brankley a claggy mist with fine drizzle lay on the landscape, dampening the vigour of spring. I skirted the field edge, close to the hedgerow. A gnarled hawthorn twig, green and lifeless, had produced many tight buds, also green, but tinged reddy-pink at the base. A great tit was alarmed, jumping from branch to branch; 'di-di-di' was its repeated electronic call. Nearby a sycamore had brown winged seeds that hung forlornly as they vibrated in the wind, plump green buds around them. Feathered olive lichen clung to the finger-width twigs. There was nothing in the air apart from a pair of crows flying across the fallow field where young teasels lay, leaves flat to the soil, ready to launch their egg-shaped seed-heads into the air in the months to come. On occasion there were aggressive-looking thistles decorated with countless water droplets. From the top I looked back down through the mist, horizon enveloped and lost. A couple more crows passed by. Then dozens of chaffinches emerged from nowhere and bounced as one across the field. En masse they landed on three power lines hanging post to post. Birds on a wire, they sat still, but chattered incessantly. Half left, and I moved on, through the wooded hilltop and into another valley; another world. Always suspended in time, but more so in the mist. It was deeply soft underfoot. Rooks called in the distance, and an owl joined in. I set off back, but didn't want to leave, so looped around and looked out once again over the valley. Lines of trees, some marking out the course of streams, sank into the mist from valley bottom to distant hilltop. The mist connected me to the landscape; saturated air carried the charge. I felt my search had brought the start of a deeper connection, but knew there was more to come.

A week later, back in the village, a hanging low sun was irresistible and drew me out into the clear sky that had allowed the sun free rein all day. It was still crisp and bright as the fireball enticed me through the trees into its beam. Out into the meadow a flame of orange light ran parallel to the land, lighting only the tips of the grass and tingeing the tree tops in the hollow orange. Fifty rooks racketed over the copse before landing amongst the uppermost twigs. They were unsettled as I approached and as they rose and circled I stood beneath, head back, watching. Eleven scraggy nests before me, twelve behind. I moved on and the rooks were now over brown, ploughed earth, but returning to their roost. My return sent them into a frenzy once more, their colic cry penetrating the air and staying with me as I re-entered the woods. These rooks are rarely at peace in their tranquil home, in a copse, by a stream running through the fields. They are seldom still, hardly ever silent, but somehow live in constant harmony. Before me were two shallow craters and a pair of upended trees lying together, fallen, their wrenched-apart roots revealed. A sudden return to earth, and they were set for gradual decay.

A turn of the Earth later, the setting sun was tempered by a thin layer of cloud. No fire, no beam of light, rather a smudged and indistinct form behind the cloud, smeared from grey through orange, to wisps of white above. The water in the pools was still and a vague smoke-like mist hung above. The rooks were still unsettled, emitting their grinding shout as they glided, or higher-pitched crying as they argued. Rather than staying to observe I departed, and at the centre of the meadow I stopped and stood alone. Two horizontal orange lines stretched out behind the rookery, but today the trees in the hollows stood dark.

I was welcomed to a new ordinary place by a buzzard and a bevy of fieldfares. The lagoon at Drakelow was an airfield, where slender black cormorants flew by, with neck extended, body static, wings beating rapidly just above the water. Some carried twigs, whilst others perched in yellow trees stained white, their beaks held proudly aloft, white cheeks and grey mullet. Geese groaned constantly. Then they stopped, and the reeds were calm as a swan glided from within. A coot, head down, stalked a moorhen. On land yellow gorse flowers, hawthorn and elderflower leaves were emerging. Spring was taking hold and casting winter aside.

I returned the next day through a dark tunnel of overhanging trees, and as I approached black rooks took off in series and led me through. Cormorants gathered in a thicket of trees standing stark on a small island, like ghouls on the crown of a drowned stag, wings outstretched, symbolic guardians of a haunted world. On the other side there were the silver and black trunks of an aspen, made so by the sun. Its circular, wave-edged leaves littered the floor below, bereft of colour and moving into skeletal form. I stood in the shadow of a cascading willow, whose young leaves, illuminated from behind, hung calmly bright. A magpie took a view from the tallest, most slender, tree. Two coots fed peacefully within a ring of concentric circular ripples beneath furred buds of willow. Points of light came and went from the water. Reeds behind arched gently in the breeze. A bee bumbled by a shocking orange dogwood making a stand against the beige. Reeds on either side leant overhead as I walked silently on a path of moss lit bright yellow. With so much visual form and sonic variety for the mind there was little capacity to think about anything

16

mundane or intrusive, let alone ruminate on it. As if to prove the point, a dunnock burst into sweet song nearby. After scanning the trees beyond I found it six feet away. It continued until our eyes met, then quizzically it paused, restarted briefly, before it hopped a foot away to continue. I moved on. Thirty minutes had passed in an instant, but the turning of the Earth was not a concern. I stood in the shadow of a birch to repose, beneath a half moon. The breeze buffeted the back of my head, paper-thin bark fluttered and the occasional seed-head floated by. Long-tailed tits, unaware, danced above me, their pink-orange hue bold in the sun. As I returned past the lake, coots left a lightening trail as their wake provided a reflector for the sun. From the far side the birch that had been my rest fanned out a farewell as it stood alone.

An hour before sundown, it was still clear, still crisp and still. To one side the trees denied the sun's light on long stretches across the fields. To the other a blackbird sat on the hawthorn, backlit, an outline of light contrasting with the bird's black, like the outline around its eye. Standing at the hilltop amongst the birdsong, the ever-changing phrases of the song thrush were most salient. Finches rose and fell, rose from the long grass, looped for a little while and then fell back to the cover. The path worn through the grass was just discernible against the light of the low sun. To the east the moon was a low, large faded disk, only able to reflect, not produce, light. Barely visible gossamer web was picked out as it floated in horizontal waves, lifted by the lightest movement of air. The bit stream of an unseen skylark entered my mind at a rapid baud rate. The sun set on me and I was cast into shadow. Back along the path I re-emerged into the light, my mind illuminated. The pond lay flat calm, lit only by the reflected sky with a partial purple fingerprint of cloud. Landscape squared. The bulrushes doubled, a clone of a lone oak, moon to the power two. The cooling air chilled my fingers and I headed home, closer to nature than during the months before.

III

HAWKS

18 March to 14 April

At Dunstall a broad bridleway runs straight down from the lane, past the pool where my grandfather fished, and up into the woodland. The pool is isolated by barbed wire, but the wildlife freely explored the leaf-litter as I passed. For the first time this year the warmth of the sun was notable, as was the change when a cloud intervened in the exchange. Daffodils lined the bridleway and beyond the five-bar gate the fields roll down to the squat church of Barton under Needwood. A long-tailed tit gave rapid-fire bursts as I entered the new wood. Large clouds occupied half of the sky, spread evenly at a constant altitude as they faded to the horizon. Last year's oak leaves, brown, crisp and curled, remained in position and rustled in the breeze. The warmth had brought out the butterflies. A mighty beech tree stood before me, trunk rippled like the forequarters of a bull. The trunk was silver-green, slightly pimpled with taut horizontal lines, some folded like flesh. In places the bark was ripped apart; lanced, scarred and rough, like a satellite image of a landscape. The tree stood motionless, silent and huge, but very much alive. The mightiest life standing on Earth, a real wonder when looked at afresh. A squirrel bounded across the field from the copse opposite to within a few feet of me where it stopped as our eyes met. I flinched slightly at the prospect of being mistaken for a tree, the squirrel retreated in horror and then quickly passed to the rear of the beech. In the copse a jay screamed. Nearby many pigeon feathers lay some way into the field, but there were no remains. Several yards away, amongst the new trees, there was another cluster

19

of feathers, pigeon once more, but again no carcass. On my way up and along the bridleway I had seen three further explosions of feathers in amongst the sheep and lambs and I suspected an aerial rather than land-based assault. All five were in a 200-yard line. There had been a couple of peregrine sightings a few miles away and the nearby pylons provide a useful high point from which to stoop. I don't have the dawn 'til dusk dedication shown by J.A. Baker in *The Peregrine*, but I resolved to return regularly in the hope of confirming my hypothesis with a sighting or perhaps witnessing the stoop of a peregrine.

I returned with Leon at dusk the next day and many pigeons were taking a chance above the open fields where a further set of feathers lay. We sat under the mighty beech and watched. In the woods, a little walk away, we found two more sets of feathers, one with a neatly cleaned bone between intact wings, stained with blood. There were no teeth marks on the bone and we suspected a raptor.

Once again we returned to the bridleway at dusk and saw a new addition to the splurges of feathers in the field. A buzzard-sized bird flew low from our side, its wing-beat carefree and lazy as it crossed the field of remains into the copse. Leon thought it was a buzzard, but I felt it had blue-grey wings. The sun was already sinking away behind the hill, its work done on the warmest day of the year so far. Flocks of pigeons began to appear, some flew by, many settled in the copse. We walked up to the mighty beech and joined the roost, watching each passing pigeon, awaiting drama. The trees were black, grass a deep green and the bare earth had an added red hue as the light ebbed away. We set off home; grey clouds were coming to dampen the evening fire. Brighter sky marked where the sun had departed and the church steeple stood dark against it, its flying buttresses forming the base of a rocket ship. Darkness was reclaiming the landscape and bats were reclaiming the air.

On the fourth day of the hawk hunt, Isla was keen to have a tour of the pigeon remains. The sun pushed down on the bridleway, the ground crisp, air dry, the heat reminiscent of summer. En route, my attention reverted to ordinary things and I stopped to examine the elongated bronze and silver buds of a beech, then the tight red buds of a lime. There were flecks of white on distant ploughed fields as gulls gathered, whilst some swirled above. The trunk of the mighty beech was painted by the crisp shadow of its own branches. Two squirrels spiralled rapidly down and around in pursuit. Sheep and lambs dozed in the fields with jackdaws dotted amongst them as the rooks in the trees beyond complained. A refreshing breeze was a thermal comfort rather than a reason to zip up tight. The cloud grew with the day and by sundown there was a continuous sheet of purple blue cloud patterned like a tortoise shell to reveal gaps of sky. Then an intense burning sun appeared, too bright to view, burning my retinas and a trace in my mind. The burst of light was matched by a burst of my emotions, my attention drawn to the brightness I wanted to view but could not. All I could glimpse was my slender tree, which stood amongst burning flames.

At Kedleston, the great bare oak leapt out in three dimensions providing little cover for the jay's brevity. Bright egg-size buds waited to hatch on the exhausted horse chestnut. Close by, wood smoke from the sawmill flavoured the air as a wren silently explored the woodpile before seeing me and alighting elsewhere to raise the alarm: man in the woods. It then went off to sing, but their song is not for us. Nor is the robin's song that flowed from a tree beyond. I filled my lungs with tree-filtered air and emerged by the lakeside for a double dose of solar energy, which the black Dexters beside me soaked up too.

Returning to Dunstall, the ball of fire that had bathed in blue all day was trapped behind a sheet of ice as a crow rested in a collapsing oak. Thirty scattered pigeons appeared overhead, high and random, unusual in their lack of direction with no coherent form. Some flew on; others went to their roost in the copse. They were confusing and difficult to follow. A lamb was loose on the bridleway and a posse of other lambs ran up and down on the opposite side of the fence until the errant lamb found a route through to the other side. They gathered at the base of a tree whilst another group bounded along the far field boundary and returned at pace, like a children's football team clustered around the ball. A second confusion of pigeons arrived. The lambs stood still and watched as I repaired the hole in the fence. A third swirling random mass of pigeons passed over. I walked on in an unfruitful search for new remains and reached an expanse of grass almost the size of the sky, bar a single oak. The orange shining opposite was topped by a single chunk of cloud. High altitude winds had stretched the thin cloud into silver threads that reflected the colour of the sun. The mighty beech was free of shadow and beyond the centre of the copse was a dark place full of bird calls. I walked through the half-light into the other place between day and night as the whole sky grew red. The lambs returned to their mothers and I returned home, the cool air taut around me.

After the recent extended warmth there was a mismatch between my external and internal world and my expectations were not met; the day for once was a disappointment. The abandoned cooling towers nearby faded into the grey sky that lacked any definition, it just was. The only thing with any edge was the cutting wind, slashing the mild conditions away, a handbrake on progress through the season. Narrowboats provided sound and motion as the wind whipped up lines of Morse code in the ripples which spelt out SOS – save our spring. Then a squadron of house martins from Africa appeared to provide aerial support, their rapid call like machine-gun fire. They soared, spiralled and dived down to water level in individual sorties with occasional bursts of rapid wing-beats before skating, fixed wing, in the sky again. Their sharp turns were like a water skier accelerating for a jump, a roller-coaster ride I'd like to join. Isla and I stood transfixed.

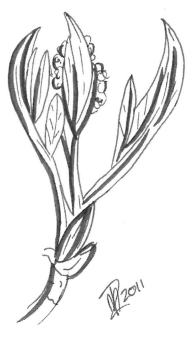

Another day and I travelled to Blithfield. Here, from a short distance the woodland had the merest hint of green as leaves began to emerge from their cramped buds. There was also activity in the fields, ploughed and harrowed to a tilth and coated with lime. Pasture striped by the roller. The most advanced buds on the sycamore felt ready to let their inner contents burst out. Rust-coloured miniature leaves surrounded an inner bloom coloured green, whilst buds nearby remained tight. Emerging rowan leaves arched up, forming the most elegant trophies. A sycamore sapling provided fresh green individual canopies and the trunk of a birch stood bold behind. Further into the wood in a more sheltered spot the sycamore were more advanced and approaching full leaf, a canopy of red-gold colour lit by the featureless sky. Bunches of bluebell foliage sat in the leaf litter, new life in old. A woodpigeon wing provided a reminder that this is a hunting ground too. As the trees turned to pine, the bluebells faded and time seemed to be on hold as I looked towards a mesh like green haze. A sole cormorant flew low across the expanse of water as three gulls repeated their comical utterances before returning to their familiar seaside yelps. The water was as smooth as the sky and the gentle wake of a lone coot painted a shimmering ever-changing curved V shape. There was a deep and fulfilling calm.

At Dunstall the next day a subtle early evening mist moderated the sun just enough to allow direct viewing, a perfect circle of yellow, lacking the power to cast a shadow and the warmth of the day had gone. Lamb 31's life had gone too; it lay moulded to the contours of the ground beneath the oak as a tractor motored back and forth, rolling the pasture. I wandered on for a little while as the sun's height and power diminished further as its size and colour increased, an orange disc hanging behind a line of oaks. A treecreeper worked the final oak silently before picking and rustling leaves caught in a pile of twigs lodged in the uppermost branches. Nearby, the blossom of the blackthorn sat bright, five white petals surrounded long stamens, each topped with an orange ball. On the same stem, some white spheres sat tight. Near the site of the woodpigeon wings I had discovered days earlier, I passed larch presenting their raspberry-filled cones of green. As I moved on, a large blue-grey bird floated down from a perch and glided through the trees in a long arc. Despite its size it was silent, stealthy, unlike the woodpigeon that seems unable to progress without noise, even in straight flight. I doubled back to follow, towards the jackdaws clacking in their roost. The bird was perched with its back to me; it turned its head and, seeing me, drifted off again. I climbed over a gate to follow, my clumsy progress frustrating me as I blundered noisily along the narrow overgrown path. I disturbed a pheasant which emitted its ridiculous blast-off cry, like a cheap child's toy on a spring. I circled again, silently, along broader paths, and passed a new circle of woodpigeon feathers below the hawk's original perch. I saw nothing more, but returned through the dampening air, exhilarated by the hunt.

Days passed and at Anslow Park the pool that was still and doubling the landscape was in motion and sending diffuse ever-changing beams of light direct to my eye from points all over its surface. Drowned long grass lay flat, calming the surface of the raised margins, looking like the filaments of a microscopic world. The wind was as powerful as the sun, cancelling out its warming effect. Nature flexed as I pushed through, past birch trees decorated with backlit bulrush fibres. A skylark rose above like a whirligig, its wings in light and shadow until it faded from view and became an audible whirligig, notes beating as fast as wings. Greenfinches rose from the hedgerow and hung, bullet-shaped. With no leaves to provide a buffer, birch twigs rattled against one another. Out of the wind the air was dense and warm; the three- and two-petal cherry tree blossom surrounded me. On and up the path, the catkins were large and pollen-yellow, the buds of the ash still matt black and lifeless. At the hilltop the air demanded to be breathed and exhaled, the external and internal worlds combining. It was a bullying wind that forced its presence on me, it took on all comers as cloud shadows rushed by. The wind ripped past my ears and danced on my hands, leaving my mind in no doubt as to where it was. As I moved into shelter, the sound of the skylark returned to dance in my ears and the warmth of the sun enveloped my hands.

April, and the head of a dead coot lay gracefully to the side of its body, the final movement of a ballerina in glistening black. There was a mixture of brightness and grey cloud as we discussed the identity of the mystery assassin. J.A. Baker had cast a poetic and literary spell on me with his account of the peregrine, and it had been a huge coincidence to find multiple plumes of woodpigeon whilst finishing reading his book, *The Peregrine*. I'd been reassessing the evidence following my sighting a few days ago. The size of the blue-grey bird led me to listen to the call of the goshawk and today we were convinced we heard it in the distance – although it is similar to that of the sparrowhawk, and even the green woodpecker.

We walked through a plantation at Dunstall attempting to identify the various trees before reaching a viewpoint. The pylon towered above the more distant church, monuments to electricity and faith. Although I'd rather they weren't a feature of the landscape, the pylons have a certain grace and today their cables matched the strata of the grey clouds beyond. A multitude of bird calls that would test all but the most well–practised birdwatcher surrounded us. A pair of black crows flew large against the deep grey cloud as the wind whipped up. We entered the established woodland towards the bridleway and Leon spotted a bluebell, advanced and alone, but for the sweetness of the primroses nearby. "They smell like beer," decided Isla, which suited me just fine. The second plantation was green, but the ash stood in a winter stupor. To the bridleway and we were all stopped in our tracks by a goshawk-like call close by. I played my guide version and it was a convincing match. Then we heard it again, in a triangle of established woodland. And a third time, perhaps fifty yards away at the most. We scanned the trees, but saw nothing. Then high above the trees soared a large hawk – not a buzzard, we are used to seeing them. We lost it into the sun.

That evening at Drakelow three lines of cloud headed from the sun towards the horizon where a series of clouds floated with perfection. To the west a line of rounded cloud fell until it formed a snowy mountain range on the horizon. Crows swooped with grace, a buzzard was perched in the birch and eight two-tone magpies squabbled in the fallow field. I glimpsed the lagoon, now curtained with green, as I headed down the hawthorn tunnel with its carpet of white blossom. Rabbits scattered across this human-sized burrow. Most of the cormorants remained tree-bound as others circled above, wings fixed until their final approach when they glowed silver in the low sun. Their chatter was constant, like a school playground. A dozen cormorants circled and landed together. The orange dogwood had burning copper flames all over. A chaffinch sang the orange-tinted evening in from a birch. With the blue sky tinged red to the east and gold to the west I felt as if I was on a jewel floating in space.

We retraced the route of the previous day at Dunstall, drawn back by the hawk of hawks. We discussed the chapter by Sir John Lister Kaye in *At the Water's Edge*, where he had an unnerving eye to mesmerising eye encounter with a concussed goshawk. A buzzard gave us a fly-by as it headed purposefully for a tree where it vanished as it perched. Then we heard what we had hoped for, the goshawk-like call travelling some distance through the sunlit air, emanating from the woods of yesterday's sighting and carried on the breeze across the rolling contours. Having progressed some distance we paused by the dead oak where we had been thrilled by a pair of buzzards several weeks before. This is a peaceful and ambient environment, soaking in nature's glory. Onwards we reached the site of the pigeon kills and previous sightings. By a gate we waited, a new woodpigeon kill in the field behind us. Leon spotted a bird land in a snag oak a couple of hundred yards away. We suspected it was a buzzard, but kept watch, hoping for confirmation when it returned to the air. We waited for some time. Then from five o'clock a goshawk flew by, perhaps twenty-five yards away, some thirty feet off the ground. It then arced to the right along the edge of the trees. I had my camera set for the suspected buzzard taking off and managed to capture the hawk. A blurred image, but enough to remove most of my doubts.

To Dunstall once again under an inverted sky of cloud – looking from below it appeared as when viewed from an aircraft. Elsewhere there were silver-blue and slate-grey stripes of cloud converging down to the horizon over the Trent Valley. To the west a fissure in the cloud shone yellow. The sheep were lambing and one lay on its back, legs in the air. There was a distant familiar call and some way on it became clear and close. I skirted the plantation boundary towards a small copse, wind roaring through the trees, shark-shaped, shark-grey cloud beyond. Was I the hunter or the hunted? Then for some unknown reason I looked right: a pair of hawks floated over the crest of the hill, steady in the wind, wings kinked as they moved closer together before they sprang apart, magnetic poles unable to meet. My mind was tuned, eyes ready for hawks light to become neural in my mind, to be given meaning, to create an internal mental representation of the external world. To create a hawk inside my mind. My keen expectations were opening me to a top-down bias, to see a hawk where there was none, but I was aware of this and resolved to confirm my sightings. These were buzzards. I entered the woods, ready to fly through the trees, densely packed upright trunks providing a slalom the goshawk could navigate with aplomb. My presence, like the hawk, caused the woodpigeons to scatter. The upper reaches of the bare trees, swayed and the branches clattered: it felt like hawk country. I was brought to my senses by that call again, in front of me. I carried on until the call came from behind, teasing me. I headed back to see a ballet of three crows hassling a hawk above the trees. It lunged at one crow before disappearing from view. I headed back, heard a further call, and then paused on the bridleway. Dozens of woodpigeon left the large dense copse. I saw nothing. The ever-changing sky was blue, deep grey and wispy white with a burning orange element. Captivated, I wanted to stay, be captured, but I had to leave this elemental place. The prospect of an extraordinary hawk had distracted me from my search for ordinary things.

It was the end of the warmest day of the year and past seven it was still glorious as we took our now familiar walk along the bridleway, through the gap in the hawthorn and around the edge of the plantation, before climbing the gate into the bluebell wood. It was very quiet compared to yesterday and we headed for the highest point of the estate. A keen-looking birdwatcher approached and we discussed hawks. He was a local and hadn't seen anything more than a sparrowhawk here, but he found my blurred image somewhat convincing. We discussed great grey shrikes and barn, long and short-eared owls circuiting simultaneously at Willington Nature Reserve. I'd always longed to see a barn owl. By now the sky was a spectacle and we headed home, dusk very much descended, through the cold air that sits at the bottom of the bridleway. We drove down the lanes and rounding a corner, there on a fence post, sat a barn owl. I stopped opposite, little more than eight feet away. It sat with its back to us, and then turned its head to take us in. It was much smaller than I expected, a delightful kitten of a bird. I lowered the window and it jumped and resettled, front-on, staring calmly at us, eyes like stellar black holes drawing in our attention. We were too close to the event horizon to avert our gaze as photons from this wisp of an owl, as beautiful as any nebula, hit us at light speed, engraving the perfect sighting in our mind's eye.

I left Needwood to connect to a contrasting coastal landscape and escape the hawk that was distracting me from my search for ordinary things. En route, the mountains of Snowdonia were just three watercolour brushstrokes floating in the haze above the horizon. At the coast, even in the evening calm, the abrupt change of landscape fired neurones that had been dormant. A new chemistry rushed through my mind. The sea fell away to a vanishing point, taking my vision further than it had been for months. The air was cool and moist despite the warmth of the day and revealed my breath, taking my inner self into the landscape and renewing my soul as the sun sank without the merest hint of fiery protest.

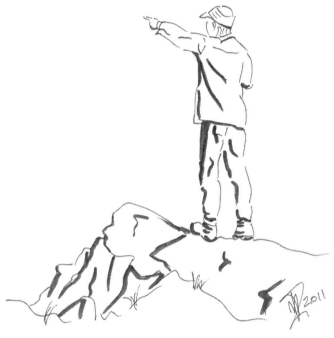

The morning was as calm as the evening before, the flat sea livened by a thousand points of light, passing through the air scented by stranded seaweed and full of the sound of the sea lightly beating the rocks that tilt back from the water, grey tan to black. Oystercatchers cried, short-lived Catherine wheels coming to a halt, joined by the sorrowful Gaelic lament of the curlew. Languid herring gulls spiralled over the bay as others called in despair as time tried to stand still. Walking along the cliff-top, there were bursts of yellow gorse flowers against the teal-blue sea and outcrops of lichened rock needled the sky. Here the sea was unsettled as currents met; a container ship out to sea sounded its deep horn. Nearby, the crisp lines of the wheatears, grey and black arc of the wing, peach breast and black eye line. We reached the ruins of Porth Wen brickworks and paused by the rocks softened by shaggy lichen. Gulls and jackdaws were on the cliff faces, and primroses and buttercups clung on above. Later I stood watching the modest swell break onto the small polished pebbles at Cemanes and a flock of thirty pied wagtails came to feed, their group flight patterns akin to their individual manner – tail wags, bird jumps, flight bounces.

Next morning rays fanned out in a mottled sky, reflected by a cliff-top pool backed by a standing shard of rock. Nearby a wheatear also stood looking out to sea. A jackdaw moved from post to post, with a grey snood and white eye bereft of empathy. At Ynys Llanddwyn, barcodes of pines stood against the bright distant hills. The old lighthouse sat abrupt, with human angles, painted white walls being reclaimed. On the beach beneath the lighthouse the sea breathed gently, we rested and the children paddled. It was the third consecutive unseasonably warm day and people were bathing in the sun and the sea. In a sheltered spot the sea held its breath, flat calm with the mildest ebb and flow; reminiscent of a highland loch. That evening herring gulls spiralled in the bay and from a lofted vantage point I was able to watch their seemingly effortless flight. Juvenile gulls appearing as accomplished as their elders. Around the headland a subtle peach sunset flavoured the still water. The sun dropped behind distant cloud, only made apparent by the sun's passage.

After three days of open skies the sun was locked behind full grey cloud, but I was ready for the change. The bay was transformed, cold, damp, windy and invigorating. The gulls still circled and oystercatchers called as they flew stiff-winged, their white wing bars and rump stark against the olive brown mass of seaweed. Towards the south stack, the weather front ended neatly, a grey eyelid moving aside to reveal a pale blue iris. The puffins had returned, although they still spent their time at sea, but I soon heard the clashing ball-bearing call of a chough rising and falling above the cliffs, home to many guillemots below. Later a pair floated for some time above us, their blunt-feathered wing tips and talon-shaped beak apparent. Up above the lighthouse swallows and house martins rocketed and weaved in the constant wind. A raven floated back and forth along the cliff-top, on occasion bringing its wings in and rolling upside down in what seemed an enjoyable romp. Back down on the beach a rocky outcrop was covered in clinging vivid ochre lichens that mapped out continents on some new world. The outcrop was also home to a single plant with eleven pink flowers, petals shaped like the beak of a chough; a hardy soul as impressive in its own way as the outline of Snowdonia behind. A swift two pints of ale meant a rush to catch the first sunset of any colour since our arrival here. On the headland opposite, four final orange reflections stood out below a turmoil of grey shower clouds tinged pink-orange. A brightly outlined fingered cloud grabbed out at the falling sun as the wind protested across the sea, which was dark and choppy up to a distinct line at the horizon where a dark cloud dumped its contents.

In the morning the sea–sky divide was still linear perfection. White wave crests faded in and then out as far as I could see. At Moelfre a torrent of white water launched on to the grey pebbled beach. It was a light refreshing steel grey, an ideal companion to the bright blue-grey sea on which two dozen gulls floated. The torrent launched through the air, trapping it in a white mass of spheres that danced in a happy turmoil around a seaweed-green rock. The stream then split into two sparkling channels before rejoining to curve neatly right then left down to the sea. From the right came a rush of sound, almost masking the more subtle splashing before me. To the left the breeze caught my ear. I had always thought I needed to live by the coast, but on hearing a robin sing I realised the simple joys of home, locked as distant from the sea as one can be. The change of heart was reinforced by my search for ordinary things in my simple landscape.

So inland and up the miners' track on Snowdon. The grass was still tired and pale from the winter and the water of Llyn Teyrn appeared black. At Llyn Llydaw it was peaceful, almost silent, when the wind dropped, the individual droplets of water working their way through the stony shore could be heard, as could a distant stream. On to Cwm Idwal, the hanging valley. Cloud gathered behind Devil's Kitchen, but it was still bright as I set out. The gnarled rowan by the bridge that I had enjoyed on previous visits was gone, lost during repairs.

Up past the mountain streams to the water's edge. Whilst I adore this place, it can induce a certain melancholy. The pyramid-shaped Pen yr Ole Wen dominated the view to the north east as the gunmetal grey slabs lay obliquely behind me. Once beneath them, surrounded by 270 degrees of steep sides, the term amphitheatre belittles the power of this place. The open end revealed blue sky, but there was no sun here and the wind blew cold. I tucked myself in, away from the wind, up by a six-foot waterfall looking out at the dark pyramid mount to the left and onto the sloping slabs to the right, the place where my father learned to climb. It started for him with a school trip to Snowdonia in 1947, which made him think about the big rock faces, and in 1948 aged 14 he returned alone for his first rock climb:

"Idwal Slabs where many young persons climbed, the Ordinary Route up the centre of the face, easy, good holds which led up to a traverse about 200ft then a steep wall above. I had a pair of boots by now with climber nails in. My memory of that day was that the boots must come off in order for me to climb the wall above me, so up I went with boots around my neck, this was hard and took me quite some time. On descending to the valley I looked up to where I'd been, I couldn't believe it."

This awe and mastery of nature is also part of our innate connection to it. I gripped the rock and thought about a description of my father's rock-climbing style by a long-time friend of his:

"He had a way of calmly assessing the next pitch and then, just as calmly but with a grip that looked as though it ought to crush the rock, smoothly and steadily ascending."

It felt good to hold the rock here, the rock on which my father had depended, to be connected like the birch that clung to the boulders above the stream where the rowan once stood. The landscape is a cue for memory and connections across time.

A day later and we were just seeing out time whilst a band of rain passed, the sole occupants of the car park at Church Bay. From this mundane setting we watched a peregrine swoop down vertically towards a crow at ground level, before rising in an arc and swooping again several times. During the display it showed its upper and lower sides following each turn, a dark upper side then lighter underparts with a darker head. The performance, for that's what it seemed to be, was reminiscent of a stunt kite diving to the ground and pulling out at the last moment. Then somehow, without moving, the hawk disappeared from view. A little later, like a bat logo hanging above a terrorised city, we saw a hawk-shaped silhouette above several gulls. It stayed apparently motionless before stooping down straight at a 45-degree angle towards one unfortunate gull, before flying off over the headland.

Gentle ringed plovers were conducting a quiet investigation of the seaweed with no fuss as we set off the next day to return to Church Bay in better weather. The clear pools were still in the smooth wet silver sand and, as I walked, a reflection of the sun in the clouds was always a few feet ahead of me. The cliffs around the bay were tall and bright and the scene for much engaging activity, a pair of ravens danced along the cliff-top, repeatedly back and forth, before taking their acrobatics high above. Groups of jackdaws argued over twigs as fulmars sat on the nest whilst their partners made numerous swooping approaches before finally landing. A pair of buzzards circled, then tangled, feet to feet. Later, at the end of our week in a different landscape, I stood on the headland as a sheet of low cloud stretched away into the distance like the sea, as if I was between the pages of a closing book.

IV

CONNECTED

15 April to 5 May

The warm weather of that week had brought about a discernible change in the Needwood landscape. The horse chestnut and sycamore were suddenly established in leaf. The woodland floor was knee-high in vegetation. The path I should take was clear, but I wanted to immerse myself. Away from the coast it was a sea of green. I felt in the thick of it, swimming through the greenery, wave upon wave of foliage. The green was now a comfort, but it can become deep and oppressive. Just as winter can be consistently stark, summer can be overwhelming green. But these spring greens are most varied, as was the birdsong in the thickening canopy.

I could not resist a trip to the hawk wood at Dunstall. As I walked down towards the pool I was welcomed by the twelve chimes of noon from the church. The sheep with their newborn lambs were sleeping in the half shade of the oaks, which were just emerging from bud, a scene described by the words of a traditional Gaelic Waulking Song I like to play: Dh' èirich Mi Moch Maduinn Chèitinn. I watched as the shadows of the occasional cloud swept across the fields that roll down towards the flat Trent Valley. In the ash plantation the tight matt black buds were being forced open and below one, there were the wing and tail feathers of a pigeon; what blood there was baked dry. This was the first kill I had found on this higher ground, but not far from previous sightings. Many bluebells were in flower, but there were plenty more to add to the show. Dandelions with their snipped and

37

trimmed petals shone yellow with the occasional sphere of those gone to seed nearby. I noticed individual dandelion seeds floating by on the breeze, highlighted by the sun, off to extend their successful claim to the grasslands. I soon realised these floating umbrellas were numerous, perhaps one in every cubic foot of air, in all directions. With the sun hidden by a branch I looked up to the treetops and hundreds of the seeds were floating past, illuminated from behind so that they appeared like snowflakes moving horizontally through the branches. The beech that was magnificent before was now resplendent, draped with young, almost crimson, leaves, a colour too rich to be described as any metal, be it copper, bronze or gold. I heard my thirteenth chime from the church and headed home.

I followed an orange tip butterfly along a path lined yellow towards a horse chestnut, a shaggy green cartoon monster emerging from the woods. The severed head of a coot lay below it, and cormorants emitted a sonic deterrent. I escaped to calmer waters, rays of early evening sunlight breaking through the cloud to light a silver foil lagoon watched over by a heron. The backdrop of beige reeds had a reflected band of green at their base. The birch where I rested was green, and nearby I heard the chaotic song of a reed warbler.

It felt like lazy summer already, with matt blue sky, flat trees, but given away by backlit cherry blossom over the ford. A blackbird sung and the church bells gave a quarter peal, then chimed nine. The willows hung within inches of the bright water of the broad flat Alderbrook. Nearby the limes made green patterns around strong branches. As I stood, mallards eagerly flew to my feet before walking back unfed. The oaks were restrained in early leaf and my slender tree stood beyond, fading into the blue haze. Birdsong was woven through the branches, interrupted by the infantile mutterings of young rooks. Once a butterfly had followed its chaotic path, travelling whilst moving, all became still in the old orchard, shadows fell comfortingly on the long bright arching grass. I moved on to recently overlooked haunts. By the pool at Anslow Park the once sodden earth was baked hard. I heard a willow warbler and brambling, before a bumblebee got inside my skull. By mid-afternoon, the air had the dense feel of summer, it had to be devoured. It was high summer transplanted into April. Spring had been squashed and uncoiled with rapid abandon. I'd been unable to keep pace with its all-round assault; I was a time traveller.

During an evening escape to Dunstall, the sun was low and warm through a distinct haze, with just a hint of cool air. A squirrel skimmed over the path as I entered a large field, home to a few hundred lambs, with fine white coats, backlit for effect. The oblique angle of the sun revealed the calm undulations in the field, and the curious lambs examined me, but soon scattered as I approached. Through the first wood and the light was deep and thick, tinged with bluebells. I stopped and all was static. Out into the open, sunlight flooded down the hillside, flowing over the tussocks of grass turning them into sunbursts, exploding from the earth all around my feet. Lifting me up towards a faded blue cotton sky. The mass of dandelions was punctuated by a dot to dot of seed-heads illuminated by the sun: a seemingly binary state, either in flower or in seed. Yellow suns and white dwarfs, lacking the breeze to go supernovae. A single shaft of light found a direct route through the wood and I was a shadow on the hillside, a barrier to the sun's projection. Looking back from the hilltop the sun was now burning behind a silk screen. The valley below was an arcade of bird calls, rapid-fire battles, phasers set to stun. But there was no sign of the boss. Just a wannabe crow on the only bare uppermost branch.

Three oaks stood in the clover and glided past one another as I walked towards the rookery wood by the Alderbrook. Out in the field there was less to process than the 360-degree onslaught in the woods behind. The rookery was more peaceful and contented than it had been, and the nests were still visible in the young canopy. The woodland floor was feet-deep in cow parsley and the route to the shallows where the children had paddled was hidden. I was a field away from where we had seen the interstellar barn owl and I felt the release of escaping hawk country to return to these neglected haunts. The field where I had found the dead buzzard was brown, ready for sowing. The lone chestnut stood on an island of green. I returned and a pair of partridges, heads like periscopes above the long grass, zig-zagged through the field to escape me. Beyond, the scattered remnants of a pigeon lay across the fissured continents of earth, just feathers and the breastbone.

The next day, at the quintessential Springwood, light dappled through young leaves and a floor of bluebells dropped away through the birch to the steel-blue water beyond. The foreground was bright, with distinct shadows rested across the water, before the birch trunks shrank into a hazed perspective. On each side of the path shards of bright grass rose pointedly up, a barrier between the massing armies in blue on either side. In a clearing six birch stumps, a few feet high, stood together by the water, calm, yet busy with sun-friendly ripples. We returned towards the sun and the young oak, birch and ash were salient to the eye, like splashes on a canvas; a natural and dynamic Pollock changing with light by the hour and by day with new growth.

I returned to Springwood the next day and sat surrounded by bluebells, birch and oak as far as the eye could see in each wooded direction, bar the glint of the water through the trees before me and the sky above. A sky building high cloud in the east: white, bright, massive and expanding. Tops towering above the trees, a slow-motion avalanche. The light was adding magic everywhere it fell, birch trunks, flowers, water and clouds. A breeze cooled the balmy air, circulated the scent and birdsong, and then draped it over my skin. I lay flat and sank into the earth, a second dimension underneath the third. In it and almost of it.

Human activity has dressed the landscape for many years. Today in the remnants of the long decimated Needwood Forest an ozone-laden smog provided a veil that flattened and diminished the trees. They sat like heavy green burdened clouds on the horizon. A close council of rooks was gathered on the scorched bare earth and the fields that were utterly sodden were baked hard, fossilised footprints marking the way. The ditch that had become a deep brown stream was not even damp, a torrent of nettles stood untroubled. The sea of dandelions beyond garners no respect, no visiting hordes, but provided its own galaxy of suns. The young birch that were bejewelled by raindrops in the winter were now fresh, their leaves fluttering with excitement. Beyond the wood into the other place even the ancient oaks were fresh and green. Where the cattle watched by the pool of floodwater, all that was primeval was a ghost tree surrounded by green. The bluebells were spread across the oak pasture, out in the open, gathered around trees like perennial confetti around a steadfast companion.

The transformation at Pool Green Wood was such that I wasn't sure of my way. The treacherous mudslides of December had been replaced by tunnels of green. The young oak leaves grabbed me, varied in form, a million juvenile decorations made by children, unblemished and inconsistent.

41

The skylark that had previously brightened our day here was still constant. Last year's bulrushes still stood, with shaggy tops, like small limbless mammals sacrificed to the gods. A golden-bowled fungus was attached to a nearby tree to collect the rewards. Another dose of bluebells lay under the sycamore, whose leaves were a deepening green. At the summit of the risings the flat of the Trent flood plain drifted away below me, a roller-coaster of trees in profile, fading to grey in the ozone haze. Even the yellow fields of oilseed rape, bright even on the most overcast day, were subdued. The rolling Needwood plateau undulated away behind me. This is a great place to comprehend the lie of the land, the hard landscape and geography that defines the nature that clings to it. The sun made its presence felt for the first time that day: a small white disc, just visible, but too bright to view in comfort.

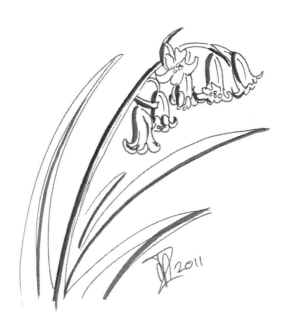

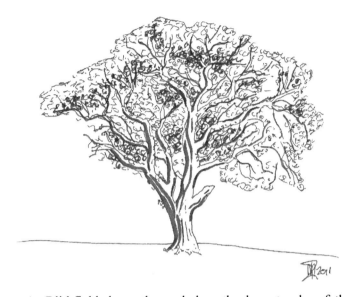

At Blithfield the path ran below the long trunks of the pine that cast shadows across the unfurling ferns. Blue sky and a line of yellow field lay behind, a linear weave of a vibrant tartan. I passed a branch of a beech, throngs of leaves dragged by the air like a willow laid on a stream. A buzzard soared above, an everyday vision and call that caused another to rise from a tree with elegant ease. It was at one with the day. A mute swan washed and rolled in the sparkling water as it preened. A crow flew low in stealth over water and then landed where a lone oak was sublimely balanced by its shadow. The beeches nearby glistened, but were dark at their core. A stroke of bluebells ran down to the water's edge where ripples focussed the sun's light towards me in a constant flicker. Returning to the woodland, individual shafts of light navigated the canopy to place selected bluebells in the limelight, lone stars in a collectivist community.

Each day changes and a white wind whipped through the hedgerows at Anslow Park, buffeting the blackbird nestled into the hawthorn. By the pool, house martins performed, flying into the wind, stalling and looping back around. The wind revealed the pale undersides of the leaves, matt, silvered green, clawing at the air as it dragged the heat out of the day. The change in conditions was as refreshing for the mind as the cold breeze was for the body. Like the wind, the cloud was in control, despatching insurgent blue to gain aerial dominance, helping April return to the norm.

On the ninth consecutive day of my search I returned to Dunstall. The sun lay long to positive affect and there was a briskness in the air. The copse was bright, free of foreboding, penetrated several trees deep by the clarity of the light. The paths were now a narrow slalom of new growth and underneath the magnificent beech I noticed that only the leaves exposed to the sun were red. The inner and shaded branches a rather limp green. My observations were interrupted as my attention was captured by the frantic alarm of two birds disturbed by a small falcon. It didn't give chase and left the pair panicking away at a tangent. The bright edge of the steel-razor sky cut down behind the trees as I navigated the blunt light of the undergrowth before emerging where the fire striker came down on the steel to give a blinding light that transformed the dandelion spheres into a thousand starburst sparks cast onto the Earth.

Today was a facsimile of a day I've known before. A day printed on paper rippling in the breeze; a dilute ink dragged across a watermarked, chromatographic sky, inks separated into their constituent dyes. It had been three weeks since it had rained, with barely half an inch of rainfall in two months. It was raining in my mind and my inner landscape was imprinted to the external world. The pale fissured earth was as crazed as the craquelure of an aged oil painting. The plain sky was a gesso canvas yearning for Turner's brush.

Yesterday the sunset had been a half-hearted brushstroke centred by a sinking droplet of orange. Today the setting sun was alone, a rocket flame departing, buffeting us with the rush from its exhaust. Trees gyrated and pulsed; grabbing, but never able to catch the wind. The slender leaves of the meadow grass bent and shone. The dandelions stood, a spent force, degenerate dwarf stars, their seeded umbrellas taken to the air in search of rain. We flew down a narrow avenue of limes, saucer-sized leaves touching across the bridleway. The hedgerows behind formed a shaggy green contrail across the landscape as we headed for May.

And May was eager and bright, a month rushing to keep up with the season. It drove across the valley floor, pushing us to Eggington and the River Dove, which lay calm, the wind only able to dress the surface with ripples that caught the light. The meadows were blown silver under the captive blue sky. This flood plain is expansive and unfrequented, feeling remote as it reaches out, inducing a flood of chemicals that blur the mind from intrusive thoughts, from any thoughts other than being connected to the river, connected with the Dove.

Time continued to rush headlong through the season, and the air was forceful once more. I tried to shelter in the lee of a stout oak but the wind gripped the trunk close, determined to hassle me. The young crops were frantic as I headed down into a large natural hollow, hoping for some respite from my new closest friend. The crops began to wave and flow with the wind, like a gently shaken length of silk rippling, the shining scales of a fish stranded on the landscape. A narrow track ran through the agitated crop and led to a lone oak. An oatmeal egg, matt and smooth, lay on the track. Forlorn in the fine dust, it tried to hold on to the light, subtle diffuse reflections revealing its three dimensions. I could not find where it might have rolled from, so moved it to the side of the path in case it was still viable. But the egg was heavy and cold, the wind anxious to give a kiss of life to the downy pheasant locked inside. By the oak tree it was calm. I could hear the wind in distant trees, a chiff-chaff, but close by a dunnock produced a torrent of delight that danced in the air: loud and unseen, but making its presence felt. Before the green cyclorama an old ash stood, scraggy and grey. A pair of swallows sat awkwardly on the path before arcing upward on the wind. In the field jackdaws fed, crows tumbled and I left reflecting on the public face of wildlife, the birds. The brave few maintaining a pleasant public image of a dramatic and hidden struggle for survival.

A couple of days later, a loaded palette knife was drawn across the evening sky, to great effect: cerulean blue, titanium white and a hint of Payne's grey smeared overhead. The sun sat, a bright pearl dropped into powder, its energy sapped and air subdued. Crows sliced from tree to earth and a sunburst transformed a pair of finches to butterflies of light as they wisped between the hedgerows. Along the path cruck-like trees formed an endless barn. The sun's glare hid the west as to the east the trees were vibrant, billowing perfection. Up towards a copse were the remains of a pheasant, attacked by an unknown aggressor, just the bones and tail feathers remaining. Inside the copse brambles had become forceful, possessive of the wood, their stiff, thorny canes arched out to attack. Beyond, the foliage of the bluebells lay spent, clinging to the woodland floor, flower stems still upright. At the exit of the wood is a stile, and I paused there for a while, in a matrix of birdsong, whose communication I could not comprehend. A mute in an overwhelming sea of messages, a desperate excluded alien. I moved on, to be met by a reassuring candelabra young beech, forming an asana of breathtaking poise and balance, its unfolding buds like candle flames. The sky was now made vast by cloud, receding and converging to a vanishing point of light. A robin stopped me under an oak tree and sang a lament as the church bells tolled eight; a plaintive, mournful and melodious piper's comfort never to be understood by me. A goldfinch shivered through the fading light and the sky was a new canvas, but I could not take any more. An evening of intense affect, visceral and reflective as one. The immersive environment was like an electric current, pulling me in or warding me away from a new dimension and level of experience. Just as my chosen landscape was becoming too familiar, I found the joy of repetition and complete connection. I felt that I had finally heard nature's voice.

V

SPANISH PLUME

6 May to 23 May

The sky was taut, stretched polymer imperfections across the troposphere. Imprinted, touched, marked; a sky used by the day being wiped clean. As time passed this celestial sphere was smoothed and slowly greyed, becoming indistinct, so that I couldn't tell if I was looking at it or through it. The trees turned to dark masses and the blackbird made its final dash, alarmed at the prospect of merging with the darkness. A tiny caterpillar on a fine thread appeared in front of my face, descending from the birch as I lay below. The robin was the last light-dweller to sing before a distant owl took over. A faint blurred crescent of moon was just apparent behind the cloud as night fell.

With the dawn chorus a volley of rain woke me, a Spanish plume arriving like a troop of Andalusian horses passing. It ceased as soon as it began, but to the east there was a new sky, with massive three-dimensional, sculpted, plasticised clouds hanging from it. The rain tried once more and soon stopped again, its functional memory erased, tentative and hesitant – unable to sustain itself. The blackbird flew above where I lay, in the opposite direction to nightfall. To the west the clouds were exiguous, meagre forms underscored with wisps of hanging grey. Unable to deliver rain, birdsong filled the void as the cooled air flowed over me. Each time the clouds tried the birch danced, but the rain could not set in. The leaves hung in forlorn fluttering anticipation, ready to be restrained by the weight of water, to hang and rest, with a constant drip from each leaf tip.

The nest-building blackbird was seeking out water and while the trees, now still, waited, she stood in the shallows. Her wings paddled the water into bright beads that fell back to her dusty brown feathers. She dipped her beak into the water and repeated the bathing before hopping out and standing still, looking as dry as when she had entered before a brief shake to ruffle her feathers and release any trapped droplets. Finished, she hopped into the undergrowth to search for food, her nest now a deep close-fitting cup containing three engaging light-blue eggs with profuse red-brown mottling.

When the rain came properly, it was solid, relentless and vertical; ideal for an immersive outing. A direct visceral engagement with the environment. The rolling landscape was bathed in bowls of moist air and in the hollows the ponds were replenished by raindrops bombing the surface, gleefully joining the caged water, mixing and creating surface bubbles and rings of bright water. By the water's edge a sycamore overhung, and the gloss green and white reflective leaves rebounded when hit. Droplets hung from the various points until tension was overcome and the mass of the Earth won the battle. The plump droplet descended to the water and sent concentric ripples forth across a few feet of water where they intersected with the smaller rings. The electric crackle of the rain on the trees all around was energising, releasing the perfume of the hawthorn to mix with the constant birdsong. We watched the low-hanging branches of a sycamore, each leaf taking it in random turn to receive a drop and wobble before becoming still again. The weight of the rain lowered the branches and we ducked along the path, drops of water running down my neck. In a clearing, nettles, pink campion, cleavers, broad leaved dock and cow parsley received the rain. We moved on to the edge of the trees. The rookery wood across the meadow stood still, subdued and cloud-like in form, but there it would be as it is here – rainfall, birdsong and subtle movement. Leon and Isla stood in the meadow, in the now heavy rain. With each surge of heavier rain my skin tightened, a primitive sympathetic autonomic reflex amplified by the reflective mind. Today the woods knew my name and spoke to me.

An unseen armada of cloud delivered a wet night, a modest amount of rainfall, but significant in that more rain fell in 12 hours than during the last 80 days. The sodden Earth was heavy and I felt leaden, pulled down to the more massive globe, static and rooted as a tree, uncomfortable in the gravity of the situation. At 4am, the pit of night, ninety minutes before sunrise, a blackbird alarm call shattered the silence. A robin then burst into song as a corvid cackle continued in the background. Whatever had upset the blackbird passed, as it broke into reassuring song.

By morning, evidence of the rain could only be seen in the dark moist hue of bare soil. However, the sky seemed to be a defeated blue and the clouds had more authority: bright white to mundane grey, they filled the void as they moved en masse with vigorous intention. A magpie traversed the wind, its white primaries sunlit and bold. We headed off towards the turmoil in the sky; an orchestration of asymmetrical and intricate cloud ripped through by an electric bebop. We arrived at Calke's wetlands conservation area, which lies unfrequented behind the rides of a pine plantation. The green corridors rise up, one with a patch of bluebells at the end a few hundred yards away, a blue bull's-eye in the green surrounds. Onwards is a stadium of tall slender trees; pine, birch, ash and even oak. Still ponds sit in the clearing between them. It is always a quiet place apart from the birdsong. Deer pass through here, we have seen them in the past, but the ground was too firm for fresh tracks.

As we wandered, Leon recalled reading *At The Water's Edge* and how he visualised the scenes, including various camera angles, but the main one above and behind the storyteller's head so his crown is visible. We discussed visualisations whilst reading and how the imagined landscape was always the same each time a particular location was described, built from a jigsaw of places we'd seen, but nowhere identifiable. We reached a wood and crossed it to a field, newly planted with several trees, presumably the aim being to create a twenty-second-century wood pasture. And, I hope, a twenty-sixth-century wood pasture. A caterpillar abseiled down from a great height into Leon's hand and above was the black boomerang of a falcon, with thin wings and a hint of a grey body – a peregrine. We watched it curve across the sky and behind the tree-line. We moved on and sat in a run-down summerhouse looking out across an expanse of grass. "I've always found swallows amazing," said Leon. They were before us, their flight like an Irish reel. Swallows and crows flew below now uniform clouds that restfully drifted and morphed as they sailed away.

There had been a threat of rain for most of the day, but through the afternoon the clouds took on a childlike representation with nothing mischievous about them. In the copse at Brankley the ferns were an unfurled elegance against the anaemic leaf litter and the light painted the ancient oak into a new form. Centuries old, but always changing. Rooks thermalled upwards and were swept onwards in the wind. The moon was a minor flaw in the blue, in apparent motion as the clouds followed the rooks' path. The trees' wooded form was apparent within a storm of illuminated foliage. Grass was shard-like, protecting the bluebells. The deep grass they nestled in was already dry, its moisture taken by the desperate dry earth. The woodland pasture was glorious, with a blue hue to each tree's shadow. The bluebells spilled out down the slope, flowing like a heady cocktail of scent, colour and movement. Floret Silva Undique.

We returned and the blackbird's nest sat tight, spiralling down into a deep home, but the three eggs were gone. Chicks of May never to be. We suspected a magpie had been the culprit. In the evening the sky conjured every cloud form possible, growing deeper and more menacing until it was enveloped by darkness, thunder, hail and rain.

The disused railway cutting was now a green vein, a canal channelling air, a tunnel of foliage. Pigeons chuffed and hawthorn blossom sat like steam frozen in time. A green artery, but not a landscape, just nature making of it what it will. It was populated by birch and ash, but the place felt abandoned rather than natural.

This sunken valley had no view of the sky and I emerged to see that it hung low, grey on grey, darkening progressively. Even the swallows were subdued as they skirted about. The air lacked buoyancy, with the swallows beating their wings continuously, rather than holding them fixed and cutting. Swifts arrived at another level, gliding with the cloud, their improbably thin wings lifting them with ease, darting along with occasional adjustments of position when a target came into sight. I left them to weave between the coming raindrops as they sank from view.

After weeks the weather system was more dynamic and the ever-changing sky drew me out as the grey disappeared and the sun set. An intense magnesium burst in a milky haze, an incandescent oxy-torch flare cutting through the landscape – a cosmic welder's flash. The low sun, unusually bright, cast my shadow upwards, painted onto the hawthorn blossom. I could not turn my head to the west; the sun was like Medusa with hair of entwining cloud. I had to position our star behind trees which became magnificent scalpel-sharp jet-black explosions against the arctic silver light. I turned away and the south was grey with a rainbow, elsewhere there was blue and silver with serpent-like clouds lying flat on the horizon.

At Anslow Park the young trees and shrubs shook whole and violently as if trying to free themselves from the earth and stride away into the unusually clear air. Together with the bright sun, I could see fine detail and true colours 20 miles away. I stood and watched a shower cloud plough across the landscape. Making steady progress, its grey curtain angled in the wind, dredging the flat surface of the Trent Valley below before enveloping the derelict cooling towers. I wondered if they are still used for nesting by peregrines, as they are regularly seen resting on the rim. As I stood, a skylark launched from the long grass near my feet with a faint click. It hovered at low level, just yards away, before releasing its song through gaping beak. Then it ascended to a great height, as though on a vertical wire, a lost angel found. Down by the pond ripples flowed between green plumes erupting to the surface. The bulrush reeds were matt green and alive. A lone swallow patrolled, skimming the surface of the water.

May had been a month of dramatic skies and today I was engulfed by a zeppelin cloud of incomprehensible size; a vast grey mother bird surrounded by white downy feathers of cloud. The fanfare of cloud became a cloak of uniform grey before it lifted to allow the sun to pierce the evening once again.

Away from Needwood at Dimminsdale Nature Reserve, a common blue butterfly crossed our path, like the petals of a bluebell taken flight and cloned with the iridescent feathers of a kingfisher. He settled and transformed a thistle whose mauve was yet to come. Wild alium garlic with white triangular flowers and petals formed starbursts above the arched leaves. Dappled in canopy-piercing light from our own star, the garlic draped the near-vertical bank in an elegant cascade. There were a few bluebells left to fly near where the snowdrops have returned to the earth. Isla noticed the large dock leaves and pink campion, touching them to understand them more fully. Ash surrounded the pond and its branches reached out as a coot jerked across with a strangled honk.

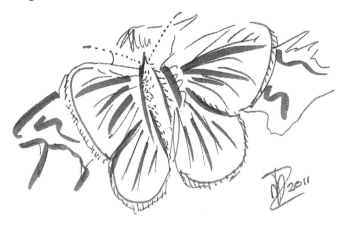

At Willington later that day, large dock leaves reached from the hedgerow offering a collection of white petals from the spent blossom. Here, cosseted between the high dense undergrowth, it was calm from the wind that buffeted above, its force revealed as I passed the field entrance. I climbed up to a viewpoint over the water to be met by an exhilaration of swifts. They bobbed on an unseen sleigh run, accelerated by the strong wind unimpeded by the lagoon, which was lit bright by sun shafts pouring through the approaching showers. The tightly clad aerial Apodiformes performed their alpine routine close to my head as a great crested grebe sat below, bemused in its fancy attire. Swift-shaped rippled light sparkled around the islands at the water's edge, before the sun was cut away and the hues of the landscape were subdued. But this was of no matter, as I was in the sky with swifts.

A juggernaut of three ducks passed through the display and I moved on along the lagoon. At the far end I stood exposed to the full force of the wind, which produced both breaking wavelets and thin stretched paths of calm across the water, like sheep tracks across a field. Inconsequential drops of rain were carried on the wind and the sun pushed through the fake shower clouds. Then there were dozens of swifts, some almost stationary just feet away from me, held up on the wind. They had a greater wingspan than I had expected, and constantly adjusted, bodies twisting, heads static with eyes always parallel to the ground. Shallow unconscious eyes that revealed their non-reflective, unaffected minds. They appeared tough and rigid birds around their flexing articulations. Even this close their bodies soaked up the light and they remained dark, with only the occasional hint of matt brown and just once, against the sun, translucent feathers of the wing.

I turned my back to the wind as rain arrived and the sunlight broke through in unison. The swifts were oblivious to the weather, seemingly capable of slaloming the water droplets. I turned into the rain and was suddenly cycling downhill through a rainstorm, the beads of water travelling bright, wind-driven bubbles rising through sparkling wine, and there was good reason to celebrate. A vast rainbow, one end dipped into the water, joined the swifts arcing through the sky, but I had already found my treasure. I felt alert and bright. The swifts were like dynamos lighting my mind, planets that orbit and power the sun. But I had no gravity, no light or warmth for them. I was just an observer passing through, an inert comet that has no impact on the surrounding witness. I was the slate upon which the interaction was recorded, the camera to the unknowing. Yet the reality did not diminish the feeling of being in the clouds and the excitement of sharing their world.

A few days later, as if not to be outdone, dozens of swallows and house martins sketched out three-dimensional trees, invisible outlines extending the rookery into the clover of the meadow, their white rumps like thistledown in a storm. It would take a million words or a fiendish algorithm to accurately describe the display. There was a constant chatter, like a falling of glass beads.

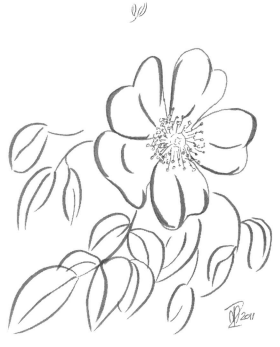

As I rounded the willows at Anslow Park, a kestrel hung in the air before me. Wings little more than quivering silk, its body was kept static and aloft, its gaze fixed on the ground below. The bird suddenly dropped from forty to twenty feet in a controlled single turn corkscrew, body vertical, gaze still fixed, before resuming a horizontal position. The decent was executed with remarkable precision, as if in an unseen tube. Memorable, controlled, bounded and compelling. The hunt was soon abandoned and I came across the bird a little while later, static once more, before moving on under a 360-degree supernatural sky. To the east, grey with an almost indiscernible peach tint towards the horizon. To the west, billowing deep clouds of grey through to white. To the north, a parting of blue with distant trails of friendly white formations. In the south, the blue continued before being surrounded by deep grey. Low, domineering, threatening – the hand of mother earth.

After a two-week break it was good to return to Dunstall, where the environment and my consciousness connected. The feeling of space was a release. The field was dotted with the detritus of lambing, two dozen pigeons and greylag geese with their goslings. The sky was silver and there was no breeze, but it was fresh enough to feel the air. I passed two fine ash standing by the pond and the fields, free from sheep, felt vast, empty and at rest. Just the jackdaw and me. I entered the woods and it was like being inside a giant organism, on a fantastic voyage. Dark wooden veins through shades of green flesh and I was the foreign body setting off alarm calls, a human splinter inflaming the wood. Stood still, the alarms subsided as the birds grew used to my form, like a needle in a meridian. I moved on amongst the brambles that blindly sought out the intruder. The bluebells were gone, their foliage faded and yellow, ready to return to earth. The only challenge to the green was the pink campion. I journeyed through the heart of the giant green being and emerged from its eye, where the light flooded in. The incoherent tune of a song thrush met me as I wandered along the trodden grass path. A fox walked into view and stopped in the long grass twenty yards away. We exchanged a good stare for quite some time. It was a young bright fox, fur vibrant and eyes reflective. It turned and ambled away, and I stopped to view the tiny red protrusions caused by the sycamore gall mite. Through a narrow path I noticed the grass move in the air, disturbed by my passing. I had forgotten just how still it was. I watched for movement in the birch and the finest overhanging grasses, but there was no motion and no sign of movement from the cooling air descending the slope. The upright fingers of new growth on the Scots pine stood above distinct bunches of green cones, another worldly alien next to the ash and wild rose. There was a prickling of thistles between me and hidden young woodpeckers frantic in an oak, whose leaves were thickening and less supple, some pale, revealing their veins. I realised my mind-occupying thoughts had gone; they had not come back, I was simply mindful that they had gone and I returned to nature, accompanied by a great tit through the young oak plantation. The sun was just a feeble pale orange stain on the foil sky as I entered the established wood, a light-consuming behemoth.

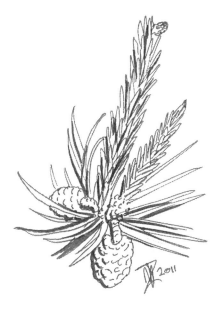

I returned two days later and noticed a tangle of wild rose in the bridleway hedge. Its grey thorns hooked down as, nearby, five white-to-pink petals surrounded yellow stamens. Although not apparent at first, there were plenty of tight buds to come. I hadn't paid the magnificent beech a visit for some time, so paused beneath it, the scene of hawk anticipation and brilliant hues. It stood firm, twisting into the earth, never to be defeated, its leaves green tarnished with crimson-brown. Amongst the erupting Scots pine were foot-high sycamore, six-leaved canopies protecting a pair of leaves below. Beyond, a chaffinch in the heart of a young oak repeated a single note that I felt in a point on my forehead. Enclosed by young ash and oak, it was calm from the grey evening bluster and I felt connected to nature, as a tree is part of a wood. The dense knee-high undergrowth gave a distinct whiff of green. The large meadow here had been left to run to tall grasses and seed-heads. I walked straight through it, as if paddling in the edge of the tide on the shore. The ebbing field revealed the invisible wind and its teasing and buffeting fluctuations, its spirit and life. The raspberry buds of larch were now plump, tinted cones, tough compared to the gentle needles. I looked up towards the dichotomous white-silver leaves of the white poplar. A gloss, deep green upper and matt, micro fibered silver underside with veins that could be read through touch. A tree within a leaf. Further on, more wild roses were calm within the plantation, breaking up the green as a symphony of vigorous ash seedlings reached up with an almost discernible strain. A bird emitted a rapidly rising sci-fi communicator shrill, but I gave no answer, for I was happy on Earth.

A torrent of sun-filled air across the evening had separated green leaves from their hosts and they had been dragged to earth. They lay curling, some cupping the day's precious rain. The hollows were untroubled by the wind and horizontal rays of light penetrated the wood so that shadows from brightly lit leaves dappled on neighbouring trunks. Sunlight reflected from the lake reached up and lit the underside of the canopy, an unfamiliar flickering sight. A harbouring beech was bright as blackbirds piloted the track before me. To think I had had to drag myself up and outside, despite my experience of unexpected rewards. The clover had been cut and the remaining grass, shorn several shades lighter, stood upright to the wind, freed from its arching load. The rookery wood appeared a dense dark green above the enlightened meadow. The swallows and martins still mapped out their path, weaving structures with invisible thread. A sight to return to, and I stood under the rookery trees looking out over the field as the birds gyrated before me and above into the blue lightly clouded sky. Looking down, a rook feather lay in the grass. It was an oily liquid underworld black with no hint of blue forgiveness. The light struggled to escape; instead it became an attached glossy film separated by a white quill that mirrored its former host's beak. As I returned home, a large cloud sat on the western horizon, punctured and ripped through at its heart. Decimated, the light came radiating through, forming spoke-like rays around the glorious hub. They extended faintly, high into the sky and across towards the north and south, forming a star of improbable scale.

VI

SOUNDSCAPES OF THE DALES

27 May to 5 June

My end of May in Needwood. Smooth gradients, cool strong air and an avenue of oaks guided my transfer into the rolling fields where fifty or more rooks blackened the cloud-filled sky that threatened both rain and brightness. The rooks noisily massed in an altogether different poetry of movement than the swallows. Despite the wind there was a settled stillness of nature just being. The breeze tried to disturb every lobe of every leaf, every stem and stalk, every twig and branch, moving around them all, causing them to clash, rustle and emit a rush that defeated the flow of air to reach me. The veteran oak had its own sound, a call of calm and knowing. Its neighbour, perhaps a century younger, has an open bole and was quieter. Watching, it was impossible to see where the sound was coming from in this unity of a million leaves. I could spend a lifetime here and perhaps part of me has, as atoms in a quantum soup of life. We have all been nature.

A fallen branch from an oak had collapsed man's boundary on impact and lay to be consumed and transformed into another entity. The track I was walking on cuts through the trees and provides a window on the wood, a deep visual field. The treetops' sway was lost as the trunk descended and the woodland floor was calm, emblazoned by lilac rhododendron. A pair of goldfinches synchronised from the hedgerow and a greater spotted woodpecker landed in the final oak just as a divorced single leaf tracked through the air, rotating at speed in a wind-curved path, to land at my feet: a thumb-sized distinctly asymmetrical runt with a compelling veined beauty when held up to the light.

I stood where the fox had stared and felt the warmth of the sun from a transformed sky. The deep, low, drawing, clasping scent of summer from the grasses arrived and left on the wind and disturbed me from my contented path. It's not so much a scent as a quality of the air. There was no trace of the constellations and galaxies of dandelions; instead, buttercups appeared to float in the grasses, their stems invisible below the yellow cups intent on the sky and rewarded with a bathing of light. Tall hawksbeard hung along the path, seed-heads, flowers and those in-between states forming a natural and rustic bouquet. Mineral red and grey cinnabar moths looked out of place, like 1980s electro-pop in the wild. A natural mascot for a decade.

Six hours later I was on a hill above Wensleydale with a new landscape of ordinary natural things before me: the fells, dry-stone walls and a run-down stone barn with wooden shutters hanging, but a fine home for a chaffinch. Below Cauldron Falls provided a new soundscape, but that was for tomorrow, as I was ready for a cheese sandwich and a beer.

I spent the night by the roar of the cauldron and by morning the waterfall was as it was the night before, sitting in an amphitheatre of rock and mature trees, beech, ash, oak and sycamore. Above, vaporous clouds moved swiftly across the window of blue that lay between the enclosing trees. The sound of the falls was a constant backdrop, almost white noise, with greater variation just audible by the more modest drops and rapids. The vibrant and varied birdsong was masked to a faint trace. Here the bird life was abundant, with chaffinch, nuthatch, blackcap, goldfinch, thrush and wagtail seen within a few minutes. Here, sound takes on the abundance of visual stimuli, an audio stream through the mind.

From Buckden Pike the water of Walden Beck comes sawing over several horizontal steps of limestone before being launched in one final extended fall onto a solid igneous pavement and then running, spent, into the deep peaty pool with its spirited Yorkshire tan. From here the beck descends a series of foot-high falls where the horizontal strata has given way. The water slows and then gathers pace over these slabs of rock, navigating boulders and riding stones. Then there is a further vigorous tumble towards the mill where man harnessed this natural force.

I took in this place; the white of the falls mirrored the sky and was reflected again in the pool at its base. Chaotic foam desperately reached up in a vain attempt to return to the brown mass of water above, some happy to descend, others desperate to return. A humble cabbage white butterfly rose to the top, like an unfurled bubble of wild water as the trees imitated the falls with a cascade of greenery. By late evening it was full of cold air and the falls drowned out the tune of the day, but not the sight of swifts in the sky above, nor the broad broken reflection of the dipper's white breast.

There was plenty to explore above the falls, hillsides of the dales and scars of rock where a looping hawk came and went with camouflage. A mistle thrush, twisted hawthorn, trees, barns and fields to explore. And we did, traversing the slopes through the lush grass, through tight stiles and onwards through sheep fields. "The king is the brown sheep and you have to walk like a soldier," said Isla. We paused to throw stones and paddle in Walden Beck, "beer-coloured" according to Isla. I was overwhelmed with the new detail making a sudden impact, rather than the incremental changes in the familiar.

At Aysgarth we walked the tourist trail and found peace upstream along the pavement of rock with its pebble-filled mirror pools. Thin coats of water ebbed onto the grey limestone, coating it silver. The river was broad, white and sun-bitten with sodden grass-clumped sides recording its flow. The broad flat flow rushed past the rocks, clinging but not wanting to stop, as material waves in a V shape deformed the surface. Forever restless, forever moving on.

By late evening I was up on the Dales again for a short stooped ascent through the scrub to Hudson Quarry Lane to scout the path to the ridge, topped by three trees and traversed, at that moment, by a rabbit. I can only attend to the detail when I know my way. The bright evening was doused by cloud along the Dale and I returned in fading light and rain to the cauldron.

The next day, cloud waterfalled over the ridge into the Dale with the wind carrying waves of hanging rain and greyness. Sheep stood in the lee of the walls as we approached Semer Water, which was choppy like a sea. "It's nice to have a wet day," said Leon. "The clouds are feeling windy," added Isla. And the wind carried the rain for so long that the sun appeared and we headed up Morpeth Gate towards a spot Turner had visited on his tour of Yorkshire. "Ooh, I like that tree," remarked Leon, looking at one of three ash trees standing in a scene remarkably similar to one I had painted from my mind a few months before. On the ridge above, a lone wind-bitten tree clung to the rock of Morpeth Scar against a steady blue sky. Running across the ridge, Hudson Quarry Lane was rutted with pathways of green between two stone walls. As we dropped down, the trees were burning in the wind. We paused to view a lapwing as a skylark managed to hold position in the wind above us. "I like the skylark song, it floats about in the air aimlessly," thought Leon. We descended steeply as the sun brush-stroked new views across the valley. We continued our descent, with ash, hawthorn and holly tunnelling us in. "Holly on the right, holly on the left, holly in the middle, holly up your vest," was Isla's view of it.

By evening it was still and we strolled out over the flat lowland of the Dale, past a farmer repairing a dry-stone wall, to where the grass was long and buttercupped. A curlew was silhouetted atop a dry-stone wall, light shining between the stones. The bird's beak was improbably long, curving down, out of balance with its body. Its call was distinctive, and together with the lapwing, filled the plain void with sounds that cut across the meadow.

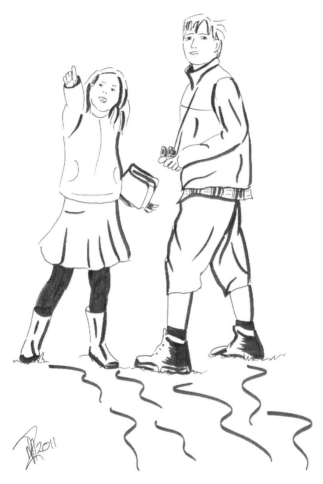

Nearby the bulbous roots of an ash spread like lava and the oak beyond were explosive frozen-ash clouds. Near where Walden and Bishop Dale becks meet we stopped, and soon saw a fish breaking the surface, a mallard with her young, long-tailed tits, swifts; together with lapwing calls and the lightest imaginable rain. In the silence we could hear the long-tailed tits grasping twigs as they flitted through the beech trees that lined this still, dark section of water which gave a sepia reflection of the far bank, distorted by ripples and occasional circles from the infrequent raindrops. Even the rain didn't want to disturb the tranquillity. A treecreeper spiralled up the trunks, its white breast lighting the bark. A family of blue tits flew from tree to tree, the fledglings calling "give it to me, give it to me", their down making them appear bigger than their parents. "See the fledgling, it's fat," pointed out Leon as it sat, owl-like, its eye markings like a slit visor.

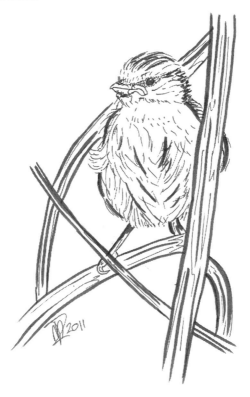

Returning, near a curve in the beck with an eroded vertical bank, we stood under a beech as the rain became more steady, but still modest. Around us was the gentle patter of the drops on the leaves, water rings and bubbles in the beck, meadows with long grasses, buttercups and birdsong. The beck had revealed the tangled roots of the trees that arch, moss-covered, into the bank. On a collapsed section of earth a clump of pink campion was bright and its reflection became indistinct in the ripples of the rain, a pink thumbprint at the end of a brush of green. Leon sat writing notes as the swallows weaved about him.

Back in the village it was the May fair, with stalls, falconry and the living tradition of the Wayzgoose border Morris side, with black and white painted faces, sticks, music and colour. They were interrupted by the hidden announcer, "Dog running starts at half past three. You'll enjoy it." I moved on, and in a nearby field a song thrush provided nature's music and then, from a sunken lane, I looked up at a blackbird stood amongst the buttercups, bold against the blue sky. Further on, up towards a forest I'd seen on the map, curlews circled and called from the meadows. I felt cupped by the Dale and peaceful in the sunshine of a landscape, generous to the eye, a new landscape to be learned and frequented. A brightness of two lapwings flew the valley as close by a curlew called from the long grass, its neck held low for a rapid clicking call and extended for its more mournful cry. I arrived back on the village green for the quoits final, a fine excuse for a pint as the sun set.

I'd been keen to visit Malham Cove. I have vague memories of visiting as a child; the beck emerging from the base, limestone pavement and disappointing photographs. Thirty years later and it was much the same. What I hadn't realised was the close proximity of Gordale Scar, and we continued our walk. It was a place where light, dark and wind battled. A place some come to conquer, many try to squeeze it into a frame, fewer take time to just be there. I was taken by the green V that leaves the scar, which was brightly lit with exceptional clear sparkling waters on tan stone. Humans have named this place, assigned their values

69

to the natural landscape. It is a scar, but a scar on the mind rather than a scar on the landscape.

Later that evening, fat on soup and beer, I climbed the dales to where the sun still shone. The sunlight raced up the hillside and left me alone, as were the trees on the ridges standing hazed against the distant muted fells. Above, the blue sky shrank to a pool of amber. The trees on the eastern ridges were crisp against the uniform blue and the curlew and lapwings still called.

June sidled in to the Dales, holding on to the bluebells at their best by catching them unawares. On the hillside twenty-three dead moles adorned the barbed wire, in various stages of decay, fur hanging scraggy, tough claws maintaining their form. A claggy grey mist hung over the neighbouring western Dale, accompanied, no doubt, by a fine rain. The low cloud extended into the south of the valley, but here it was lit bright as it enveloped the greenery. The northerly wind carried faint raindrops towards me.

The bough of a mighty ash lay slain, attached and in leaf, but decrepit. A second ash a few feet away was petrified but upright. Onwards south to the remains of a Knights Templar chapel, the sky clear and the exposed ridge becoming more wooded, with the terrace behind protected from the wind. I flushed two curlew which then started their characteristic calling and circling. As I reached the cairn on the high point of the ridge two dozen geese flew over in formation, heading east.

The next day there was warm sun, the sound of grasshoppers and flowers like a perennial border running by the river. The smell was of summer and the shade of the trees was most welcome. In the woods I came across a grey section of a long felled tree, one branch clenching a boulder tight, reminiscent of a Pompeii figure frozen in ash.

By evening the warmth of the stones in the wall was evidence of a summer's day. High on the hillside the walls had an orange tint from the sun setting on my time in the Dales. Whilst the soundscape of the curlew and lapwing had been memorable, it was the human way of life, the quoits, pubs and greens that I found most appealing.

At the falls the next morning a dipper hopped behind the water veil, the still surface below reflecting its white, in stark contrast to the deep brown of the pool. Beneath the beech, fractal-like ferns hung wide, flat and soft to the touch. Shafts of light were visible through the morning haze that sat in the deep glade of the falls and the limestone overhangs were painted with the rippled reflections from the pool; even the thick dry moss shone. Against the sun minute particles flowed and insects zigzagged whilst other particles rained from the trees. Somehow the song of a greenfinch overpowered the sound of the falls.

Back home that night I felt buried alive by the silence. Gone was the water; there was no wind and, in the dark, without senses stimulated, there was no soundscape, no landscape, no connectedness to nature. I set out as soon as I could into a summer's day. The pine trees were now deep in greenery, their stub-dressed trunks dark against the rising mass of ferns. The path was lined with the occasional foxglove and wide-reaching bramble flowers, one with eight petals reduced to five looked like a dancing figure, their scraggy form in keeping with their prickly host. "I've just seen a beautiful dark green dragonfly. It was absolutely beautiful," said Isla. Our destination was a wildflower meadow, full of red poppies last summer, and today it was whiter than the sun-drenched clouds above. A meadow dense with ox-eye daisies, like a field of corn with every stem carrying half a dozen wide daisies with firm yellow middles. Isla bounced her teddy bear across the whiteness and we left with pollen on his nose.

The next day brought a trip to the ford for Leon and Isla to catch some minnows. We'd made a trap from a plastic water bottle and left it downstream whilst testing our skill with nets. Standing silent in the water gave us a new perspective as we waited for the minnows to gather close to us as fledgling birds scattered about. This time brought childhood memories to the fore, with parenting presenting the chance to revisit the things I had enjoyed years before. I spent my entire childhood in this village. I'd spent many hours wading up and down the Alderbrook as a child, but as a playground rather than an escape. Brook Hollows was also a frequent haunt for den-building, scrambling on my bicycle and generally messing about.

Later I headed out alone as the light rain beat on the young beech around me; a world of grey and green. The sky was like a polished stone, dripping wet. A cow called out like a distressed human who had lost the power of speech – a haunting soundscape that hung in the air and then my mind.

VII

EQUINOX

6 June to 21 June

Out by the Trent, Isla spotted pale, tinged pink, heart-shaped petals of the wild rose lying on the path before us. "I wonder why they are heart-shaped?" she asked. I thought it could be that the heart symbol comes from the petal and later I was surprised to find no reference to this, although I didn't look too hard. Given that the rose has been a symbol of love since Roman times at least, and the wild rose is native across Asia, Europe and North America, it seems quite possible – and certainly more compelling and beautiful than the Freudian suggestion of the symbol being based on various aspects of human anatomy. We moved on. "That's a nice tree," said Leon. Isla swung from a low branch: "I like it a lot!" It was a squat oak with branches shooting out at ninety degrees just a few feet from the ground. Then the trunk turned into a dozen or more branches a couple of feet higher.

That evening I ventured out alone again. It may not be grand, it may not be extensive, but this simple Needwood landscape on a summer evening is so special to me, and my shadow cast across it, as the trees and birds. I was deeply affected and released. The swallow's beat, the undulating fields and steadfast trees spoke new words to me each time I arrived on my search for ordinary things. Ordinary nature is more compelling than our most extraordinary art. I walked past the trees I'd seen through winter and spring with a greater awareness of their journey. The matrix of birdsong was more simple, a more accessible soundscape. The birds seemed more content, their territory secure, mates found; or perhaps, with mouths to feed, they were just too busy. I found a recent pigeon kill, this time a ringed racing bird. Not quick enough.

Near my previous sighting I saw another fox on its regular path through the long grasses and young trees. It was bigger, darker, less willing to exchange a stare, but relaxed enough to amble away. I followed a path decorated with clover in flower until it faded and the landscape became just dark green. Later the sun found a path through the established woodland and I walked in its spotlight, projected onto the trees before me, my form travelling into the future, a ghost in the woods.

A squid of cloud inked the horizon under an ocean of cloud. A shoal of swifts danced past and the water-doused land swallowed the erupting sun.

The foliage seemed distant and harsh, buzzing around me, as today the woods could not clear my mind. I headed for the rookery in low sun and light rain. A painter's smear of grey showed a heavier downfall nearby, but I was ready to be cleansed. The rookery trees reached out across the meadow with their shadows, for their swallow weavers were gone, as too were the rooks. There was no rookery noise, just sound – the church bells, distant birdsong, movements in the leaf litter and the constancy of the weir. I stood below the deserted nests and the bells ceased. All I could hear was the light rain engaging with the canopy until, from the east, a bevy of twelve rooks passed by. Looking back to the hollows, pigeons were lifting from the meadow into the trees. I was then connected, plugged in and energised, free to breathe deeply, and the bells resumed, a full peal in celebration of my reunion with nature.

Days moved on and the grasses at Brankley were tinged with shades of purple seed-heads that broke up the expanse of the meadow, as did the cloud for the sky. A skylark provided a lone song whilst hidden, as was the sun providing light. The air was unusually cold for June; it had a winter crispness. In the meadow a succession of plants had shown and passed, and lay spent. I entered the other world of the wood. Ancient, subdued light, ferns and peaty earth. The deep gloss of beech brushed against me as I approached the veteran oak, which was, as ever, bulbous, bent. In the pasture a yard of thistle stood, topped by a purple flower and a cluster of buds. Over the valley to the west the sky was salmon as rays gave away the position of the sun. A solid calm trapped me. I was lone.

After a night, the tallest cow parsley leant in and offered its saucer of Y-petalled blooms direct to my senses. I stood near the site of our best goshawk sighting, the ground now deep in undergrowth. Close by, on the grass, lay an explosion of feathers, grey-white banded with an olive half: a laughing green woodpecker silenced by an unknown laughing assassin. I revisited the corners of Dunstall I'd not been to for several months and glanced a buzzard, flowing like bronzed Yorkshire water through the trees. Wandering through the sunshine and young trees I come upon two fox cubs being curious in the long grass. I stood silent, watching, until they picked up my scent and retreated calmly into the woods, before galloping away through the undergrowth. I set off again, through the field where dandelions had been, then buttercups and now purple ears of grass. In the rhythm of walking I forced myself to stop and take time. I held a young ash close by; its leaves were cool, as was the bark. A chaffinch sang from the wild rose and as I moved on I realised chaffinch song was all around me. I was content. I was summer.

As I left I reflected on my year-long search for ordinary things. It is, by definition, straightforward, but approaching halfway through the year, I started to consider the impact of my journey. I had found a greater awareness of change. Of variety. Of pleasure. Of interest. Of the joy in repetition of a location with its changing environment. Addiction or contentment of place? There have been highlights. Events, such as the hunt for hawks, the arrival of the swifts and swallows. And the surroundings I have found close by; water, fields, trees and sky. There are also highlights in affect: the floods of feelings as elements of nature burrowed into my mind, like a leech letting blood. Being at one with my fascination, but no less curious.

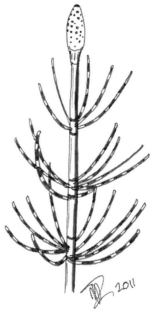

It was a day when the rain radar showed a wet mass approaching from the south-west, so we headed for the wooded nature reserve at Hilton, a favourite spot for a wet day. The grassy floor of the birch glade was so fresh that it was brighter than the sky. Close by, in the margins of the pond, were yellow flag iris, arching leaves brightly jewelled by the rain. Then there was a mass of banded horsetail, a living fossil, around since the dinosaurs I pointed out. This started Isla off on evolution, a topic I'd struggled to get across to her a couple of weeks before when she concluded that a monkey was once born with a human face. "Do humans dissolve into monkeys when they die?" she asked.

The dichotomous evening sky was stitched together by birdsong. I walked under the close hand of cloud that was edged with light. At nine o'clock the oaks were of the deepest green. The wood was in gloom. The hollows. The black bed of the stream glistened as white ripples piled and fell beneath my feet as I stood above the dark serpent that carves deep between the trees. I followed the dark veins through the woods, past ivy-throttled trunks until I found light over the lake. The reflected sun cast my shadow both up into the branches and the dell below. I could smell yesterday's rain and the woods were strangely quiet as the sun slid over the meadow and below the hand of cloud there was balance. As I headed home the hand lifted to reveal contrails across the blue. A dragonfly wing of cloud hovered over the horizon, a burning sun at its head, peaching the departing cloud.

A morning chorus started my day and a shared evening with Isla ended it. I was content before we left, but it was a sky to be shared, so complex it required a shared cognition. Up the bridleway we went, past the green woodpecker's feathers and on towards the snag tree where Leon and I had seen buzzards months before. "That's a nice tree. It looks like it's been electrocuted," Isla pointed out. Hoping to see the foxes, we waited. I leant on the fence as Isla sat on top of it with a bag of sweets. Out of the packet came 'Cool Dude' and 'Sweetheart' – you don't need to know which one I got! Isla quizzed me on birdsong and after a while we retreated: no fox, but thousands of words shared.

The green mass still expanded in a spurt of growth despite the drought. Nettles reached six feet as they clustered

77

and reached along the path that on a cycle I once roared. I reached the field to the rookery wood as the wind increased and lonely raindrops fell briefly. I retreated to the woods and looked up into the twenty-yard world between my head and the canopy. Branches reached across the green, some fallen and hanging in space amongst ivy-clad trunks. It was a rediscovered dimension accompanied by a new light. I stood in the flesh of the Earth, in the flow of the wood.

After an impressive morning cloudburst, we set off for Dunstall and searched the long grass for grasshoppers. There had been little rain here and there was warm sun between heavy grey clouds, lighting the new red leaves of an oak, their veins yellow. At our favourite stile we paused and turned to look back. A couple of fields away a filter of grey rain had descended and vapour was rising. Rather than run a hundred yards for cover, we put on our macs: a tactical error! Keen to avoid admission of this, we stayed put for thirty very wet seconds before running for cover, getting drenched in the process. We enjoyed our mistake under a tree. After the rain had passed we walked out into the plantation and found many inch-wide pink flowers nestling at ground level. "They look like circus tents and they smell so nice," Isla observed, being much more able to reach their level than I. A few yards away there were some white versions. "I think these are the same. They're just earlier in their life cycle. You can see the pink coming in," noted Leon.

That evening I stood by a field of corn, a light matt green like dry sand, soaking up the light and taking shadow. Swallows harvested close above, rapid glinting sand yachts sinewing along before taking to the air. The ears of corn shook excitedly, in appreciation.

Pink spearheads of foxglove pierced the flesh of fern that bristled with briers. A matrix of birdsong netted the wood and I was instantly connected into nature's existence. No thoughts or memories activated, just being. At the sump of the wood lies an atmospheric black pool, pierced by tree stumps. "I like this pond, it's still," said Leon. A coot and its baby came into view. "That's the first life I've ever seen on it," he continued. Moving on, Isla laughed through the tickling grass-heads that leant over the path, beckoning us on to a further wood.

Paradoxically, the coming of the extended light of the summer equinox coincides with the oncoming of the green darkness in the wood, dark apart from the young horse chestnut that fanned its broad adult leaves over the water. The ripples travelled across the lake as relentless as time, the time that will see the summer light be taken tonight and the green leaves brown and fall, but for now we are summer, sitting on the waterside.

That evening Leon and I went on a fox watch. As the cloud-hidden sun's rays fell, we crept, waited, crept and paused without fox reward, seeing only a family of long-tailed tits bending the uppermost birch twigs. We retreated in the sunshine, our conversation turning from foxes to rams and Derby County's prospects for the season to come.

I had reached equinox. The Earth was most inclined and the sky was as vast as the day was long: time stretched, perception slowed. At Willington, two angel-white swans, serene across our low bright sun, bejewelled the lake on landing, whilst ducks rowed below. A strong wind chopped the water between islands of calm that reflected the willow. And I was an island of calm. Tall grasses stood near, with their seed-heads apparently perched on the horizon like distant trees beyond the lagoon. A cloud of gnats was illuminated gold. There were languid gulls, swifts, martins, tern in the air and others of their kind in the reed and hawthorn, whose berries were stained red where they faced the sun. A bullfinch stole the robin's flair and a flight of ducks slid the fanned rays of the sun, as slowly the day submitted to the inevitable. As I returned, the power of a nightingale's song arrested my attention and entwined my heart. Agape, I became little more than a receptacle for its voice.

VIII

THE DARKNESS OF MIDSUMMER

23 June to 3 August

Yesterday's collapsed willow dying into the lake was all that spoke to me. I had reached the plateau and green darkness of summer. My mind wandered happily from the nature around me to music based in the landscape. For me, the music of Martyn Bennett is most rooted in the hills. Martyn was an inventive piper, fiddle-player and composer who combined elements of classical and jazz with traditional Scottish music, dance beats and recordings of nature. Like the landscape, his compositions were powerful, colourful and created from multiple elements, from delicate tunes around the peewit to uncompromising hardcore music that reflected the hard lands of the Cuillin. Sadly, unlike the landscape, his time was limited.

Today the grass flicked across our feet as we circuited Anslow Park. "I like listening to the birds," said Isla, they were living and jiving the world they were in as we sloped to the highest point. Looking out east over the Trent Valley, a buzzard soared towards the cooling towers of Willington. Having passed thistle thickets and seed-heads of grass, silver in the light, we sat quietly by the pond and the wildlife came. Swallows skimmed, a cuckoo passed, reed warblers called, a single moorhen patrolled the margins and a little grebe appeared, to dive and then emerge. Isla wanted a carry back; snuggled together, we walked towards the sun. Embraced by kin and nature, there was no better place to be. Not even the kind of solid grey wet summer's day I adore. Not too wet, still and infrequent.

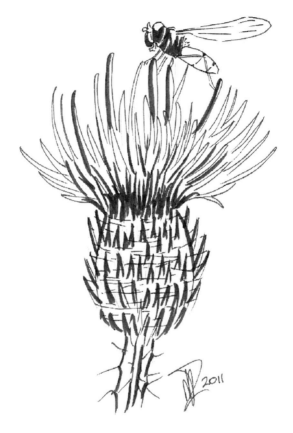

And that wet summer's day arrived. At Drakelow the Trent lay heavy and smooth in its bed, accumulating rainfall. The banks were packed with colour, foliage fading to yellow, patches of white, splashes of purple and, of course, greens. It was a wild perennial border. The smell here was reminiscent of the rabbit shed at school, a dark funky place with aggressive inmates. I bolted down the dark hedgerow tunnel crossed by briers, occupied by gnats and carpeted with damp blackened leaves spotted with ragged mushrooms. All within a dense air pulsating with waves of birdsong, particularly that of a dunnock close by. As a pheasant choked I emerged from the tunnel, sodden below the knees, to a show of vertical purple blooms. Close by, ox-eye daises and droplet-lensed pink wild mallow combined gloriously. Curved spikes, from subdued orange to a fired yellow, punched the humid air and came rocketing into my mind. I stood and surveyed the wild garden that lay below a crow perched on a snag tree as cormorants flew over the lagoon as they had done in March. There were thistle buds at all stages of bloom. Woven with delicate threads between their cupping spines, one examined and harvested by a hoverfly. Life was everywhere and I felt I was within a book's hand-illustrated nature scene, where all manner of flora and fauna comes together. By the time I left the page, the cloud was breaking and the air warming, tightening its humid grip on the day.

The hottest day of summer so far followed and, although there was a breeze, it was a day to stay close to home and retreat to the shade or lie back and watch the swifts pass. And they did, under high flat skies spanned by a fingerprint of cloud, blurred around the edges. On the clouds moved, gently rotating and changing their vaporous form, to which the mind gives meaning; a lobster, rabbit-head and whale passed overhead. Later, more three-dimensional forms appeared, lit to an alpine glare, before they too slipped away to blue. There were swallows too, collecting insects for their young in the nest above me. Flying low around the willows they spent half a minute gathering food before a rapid return to stall at the nest. Other times they disappeared for several minutes before returning. Whilst waiting a sparrowhawk passed, before house martins took their turn. Three goldfinches spirited over, and a magpie, a crow and a buzzard, before I drifted off, stroked by the breeze.

The mini heatwave continued and the thermal discomfort of a thirty-degree-plus day made my search for ordinary things difficult, but relief came in an evening change. As it cooled the wind roared, animating the trees as fish leaped in the water. Leon and I sat in the hollows, comfortable as the sun fell behind a maelstrom of grey cloud, a summer madness shooting an arrow of light across the lake. Back home, with light fading and blackbirds reasserting their claim, I underwent my final phase of cooling, assisted by slow raindrops. The cloud thickened and the rain persisted. When it was done the call of the blackbirds remained, held in the still air under a cushion of low cloud that the song seemed to describe. It ended with the blackbird's final flight and alarm call. All the elements had fallen into place for a perfect descent into the night and I remained with them into darkness, left with the distant hum of man.

Oak stood and sun shone bright on a final June evening. At Anslow Park the air was still with a slight chill where shadows grew long and ridge and furrows were revealed. The sky was blue-centred, with a white cloud surround, and birds sung through the sense of moisture in the air. As night grew close the cloud took on the pink of flesh, as the air blanched my extremities, sapping their warmth. Fingertips cold, and above, wing tips glistened where the sun still shone. A blackbird on a bare ash branch was perched in the light, its song the sound of the essence of the day being imbibed into its blackness for release at first light tomorrow.

Denied the day, it was on the cusp of night before I got to engage with July. Fiery cloud had passed and all that was left was darkness and pin-pricks of stars. I chilled under the plough and wondered what might have been. Restless, I had to retire on a day that had had no chance to draw me out.

I awoke to a surgical sky, its clinical light giving precise shadows. The horizon sky had high summer's subdued tone. Trees sat heavy and matt. The air's early freshness had left and two jackdaws clawed the sky. A bubbling of woodpigeon calls washed throughout Brook Hollows and a wren called out for fear of being drowned.

By noon the air was thick and could be tasted on the tongue as we rambled the lagooned nature reserve at Drakelow. As we headed for a place to sit, green woodpeckers shone away down the mossy track, sided by golden flowers. There were plenty of young coots and a heron on the water, while before us there was a good deal of rustling and squeaking in the reeds. We watched for quite some time. "It won't show itself. It's a private one," said Isla, so we left, ignited into action by the spark of an electric-blue dragonfly. By early afternoon the clouds expanded and shared the sky as swifts railed from blue to white and back as I dozed.

At Eggington there was a flood of crevassed cloud above the flat lands that lie to both sides of the Dove. Light shafts punched down to the flat seam of green. Leon and I walked along the banked earth of the flood defence, tracked by sheep that had left their distinct stench. We navigated the furrows of a potato field towards a disused railway embankment before returning. We paused on a bridge over the brook to watch the Banded Demoiselle damselflies. Their blue and black X-wings fluttered as they feinted and chased their reflections, before resting on stubs of reeds protruding from the water. By the riverbank there were dozens more. It was so quiet their wings could be heard as they passed close before resting on the arching grasses. We sat on the bank and discussed the sky and why fish break the surface. The water was still and heavy, apparently motionless below several clouds of manic flies. A damselfly seemed stuck in the tense surface of the water, when suddenly another arrived and pulled it clear. A black-headed gull followed the course of the river silently. It was that sort of evening. A section of cloud had darkened under its own mass, as if it was ready to collapse into a dark moon in the expansive sun-streaked sky that was above us and below us, reflected at our feet.

The hotter weather had been short-lived compared to summers past, but enough to hold me back from my longer walks. The atmosphere was such that I became aware of the interface between body and air and the uncomfortable warmth. Even though the plain, almost grey, veil of cloud subdued the sun, there was still a clinging air as I headed for the local relief of Brook Hollows. Cool air seeped out from the woods as I approached and within it was refreshing and still, with the sound of running water helping to draw away the heat. I sat at the site of the old fishing hut, two mallards in front of me by the pool, beaks tucked under their wings, docile. Two more landed in the brown silted water, once clear enough to sight bream, but the silt trap and osier beds beyond are long gone. The swans are gone too, leaving after their eggs were deliberately destroyed.

The rookery meadow had been cut a second time and the stubble was satisfying to cross as a breeze freshened the air. The unfrequented rookery wood had more birdsong, but still lone voices. The brook flowed through a tunnel of green as I stood where I had stood months before, awaiting spring. Summer had bought a different world. As I left the wood, I turned to see a large brown bird, my instant thought was that it was a buzzard, but it departed with hawk-shaped wings that quickened to the horizon. Rebalanced, curious and wanting more of what nature had to give, I headed home for the turning away.

A couple of days later I arrived at Dunstall with my mind a clear pool, as it had increasingly been. The recent heat had gone and the sky was a distant silver wash, tinged blue, with shower clouds hanging below. At the horizon there were steel-grey clouds against the silver. Above, silver clouds against a steel-grey, which was scribed by swallows. Beneath lay the remains of a magpie, forlorn blue-green oiled primary overlapping pied feathers. The purple-tipped grasses had faded to fawn on autumnal stems, reminiscent of a beach with a wave of ragged flowering clover breaking on its edge – the sound of the sea created by the wind in the trees. I traversed the grassy shore towards a more varied palette of grasses, dried and spent oils painting an unintended scene as several crows swept the treetops, their blackness seeping and staining the sky to grey as rain began to fall. As the sky changed the landscape changed – but let's not forget how our minds can change our view of the landscape too.

The sun and thunderclouds sent their light to Earth, mediated by a droplet-formed rainbow. Electric bursts of raindrops bounced on the ground below defeated and deafening grey skies. But there was also blue sky and tumbled towers of erupting cloud, an elemental laboratory of energy, light and sound coming together to concoct a new life. Then there was shadow as the sodden earth glistened. The greens changed shade and waited. And then came the wind, shadows gone. In what seemed a blink of an eye the sky had changed, rotated, inverted. Looming continents of cloud drifted, forming and closing oceans; seas navigated by jets. It was a sci-fi interstellar nursery of a sky as I left to enter the deep space of the landscape.

We thrashed our way through hunting nettles and brushed through face-high ferns that coated us with water from recent rain, but were still more engaging than nettles. "Daddy, it's a jungle in those ferns!" cried Isla as she emerged, and Springwood did feel like a different place. We suddenly left the woodland floor of green, to a denser, more mature wood with a floor of leaf litter, where birdsong was free to air. Reaching the reservoir it looked low, despite the rain, revealing a road descending into the water. A Concorde tern passed as a buzzard called. The leaves of the birch trees crackled. An avalanche of dark green descended the hillside, with brighter willow marking the leading billowing edge of the fall. The dark wood became darker as clouds and wind came, and we turned for home. Rain arrived as we parted the ferns once more, revealing the vertical forest within a forest, a wilderness within the ferns. We passed spent bluebells carrying black pearl seeds in crisp brown cups. The shovelling call of the great tit came with the sunshine, and robins conversed, just as we did.

At Brankley, there was simultaneous full sun and light rain as I crossed a meadow to the sound of skylark and grasshoppers. The grasshoppers' constant sound was matched by the visual shimmering of the young birch. Sandwiched by sound and elements I watched a bee harvest multiple blooms. I approached the old man of the wood, through ferns, disturbing blackbirds exploring the leaf litter. And there it stood, its trunk calloused, bulbous and supportive of two branches. One was hefty and approaching vertical, the other gently rising from the ground, but hollowed; rotting within, yet home to twiggy new growth. Hoverflies became light-emitting as they hung suspended in a beam of sunlight breaking the canopy, as my shadow sat surrounded by a quivering of leaf shadows. There was no birdsong, just sound from the wind in the trees, flies and distant grasshoppers from the meadow outside the wood. An inchworm before me looped lazily along, gripping with toothcomb legs, always holding one end aloft before planting itself and swiftly bringing forward its rear and releasing its fore to pause once more. I headed back through a purple and yellow bordered path to be stopped by an azure blue cornflower, with four toothed fletches piercing a purple heart.

The next day a pair of crows darkened the hollows as they hawked between the trees with uncompromising blackness. Out towards rookery wood a hidden heron took flight, reflecting the mood of the day with its calm and gentle movement. Isla and I watched a brown and cream-edged ringlet butterfly progress along the field margin, seemingly incapable of knowing its direction. "Gosh! Look at that tree," exclaimed Isla, pointing out a seemingly dead fir with a living allegro rust colour, flames amidst the green darkness. Isla wondered where the rooks had gone and then bent down to inspect the underside of a nearby sycamore leaf. "All those little bugs are there again," she said, having seen a host of greenfly. We moved on to a pool in the Alderbrook. "Look, there's a bug in the water. Just that little bug has made a huge circle, look!" Isla said, whilst motioning her arms around as a circle of bright water grew to six feet in diameter. We followed a path through the cornfield and Isla stood for some time on the stile, before saying, "I'd like to be standing here all day."

A few days before, forty pigeons had sat converging on parallel power lines heading down into the valley under a drawn gossamer sky that draped the sun, but I resisted the call to explore the day. Sometimes I have found it difficult to decide where to go on my search for ordinary things. In fact, the intensity of the search has been such that sometimes I have found it difficult to decide when not to go. Tonight was one of those nights, the first opportunity for three days. Or should I leave it for a couple more? Recently the days had seen calm and subdued weather with plenty of cloud. Tonight the cloud had broken, but as I walked up the bridleway I felt the days were repeating themselves. The progress of fresh renewal had slowed and I felt the pendulum slowing to the turn. And then a pair of buzzards captured me, moving between the trees, disappearing from view. Something seemed to be going on and I chased their plastic call through the still massing undergrowth towards the mighty beech with its crimson depth. The calls returned to where I had started, but I carried on, scratched by the undergrowth, physically, rather than mentally, attached to nature. In the fir plantation, this year's growth was blending in with that of the previous years and the calls kept on, to be joined by others. I felt the excitement of my return to the paths I had tracked in the days of spring. The memories of those days seemed fresh and, like the undergrowth, I felt like I had grown here too.

The sunlit air was uplifting, cool and peaceful; I could hear the whistle of a pigeon's wings one hundred yards distant. Indecisive of my route I headed towards the setting sun through a field targeted by a million glass fibre-like grasses all angled north, like a volley of spent arrows fallen from a great height. I felt misled and teased by the birds, which still called as I looked back on where I had been. And then as a leaf dropped I realised the spell had been cast and the die set. I was connected, part of the landscape, as a neurone is part of a mind.

A vast Northumbrian style sky shattered by the falling sun. Ox-eye daises became bright moons as the black crow surveyed.

A sheep track runs up towards the mighty beech, and today in the high sun it glistened. The air was thick and the sun warm on my skin as I walked up the bridleway. Cattle sheltered under the trees where I'd seen the buzzards two days before, but all was quiet today, apart from the breeze in the canopy. The long grasses reached and grasped my ankles as, close by, a bumble of yellow and black cinnabar caterpillars clung to their favoured plant. The grasshoppers ticked, like an analogue stopwatch reminding me of the passing time. Time; even when I set out I know I'll be compelled by time to return. Time, the regulator. A whistle from a nearby steam rally explored every fold of the landscape with its sound and I moved on. The undergrowth in the wood looked defeated, wilted to the ground or yellowing like the nettles here. The wave of purple and cream grasses caught the wind in their own manner, and I was cooled by the funnel of air caught in the contours of the rolling and descending meadow. A buzzard wired down the path before me and then veered off to where it was free to go. And I returned, defeated by space and time.

For the first time I felt like taking a break from my search this weekend. I did other things, but by Sunday afternoon Leon was keen to walk by the Dove at Eggington, where we had been two weeks before. A tentative blackbird welcomed us under spitting skies and the wind drew firmly across the flood plain. Clouds queued like tankers in orderly, even-spaced lines to bring the promised rain. We followed the bank of the river, as did a host of sand martins, scouting a stretch where banks were cliff-edged, the water audibly rapid, stretching the green weed enjoying the flow. Past an oxbow, we reached the pillars of the old railway bridge that remain, standing in the water. Making our way through the wildflowers, we explored the bank for a little while before returning. Beneath a languishing crow we reached our natural bank seat and sat amongst the swaying grasses and ripped willow. "Last time the water was so still you could see everything's reflection. This time it's blurred," Leon said, and the river was just light and shade. Downstream we watched a black-headed gull as it hung in the wind, like a kestrel, but eventually bobbing and weaving in the gale, white against the willows. "It doesn't feel particularly summery, more like autumn," commented Leon and a watery sun tried its best to rectify that, giving enough to pick out the ripples. As the rain came we sat, dry and sheltered by umbrellas, as the ringed river flowed by. I asked if anything was happening on Leon's side. "No, there are some sheep that keep staring at me, and I'm staring back," Leon replied. And there we sat, undisturbed, bar the sheep.

I felt as if my search was continuing to wane the next day as, to the north, a hill of sunlit spring green pasture abutted the deep-grey banded rain cloud as the sun set brightly to the west. We walked the woods, spent and lacking vigour; I felt hollow. Not even the blackbird could lift me. The pendulum had stopped and, working to the calendar, a summer of June, July and August, it was midsummer. Perhaps my abatement was caused by the slowing of the landscape to which I have become connected.

It was a cool melancholy day; smooth clouded bands of blue-grey radiated from the south before collapsing into a northern wall where they cleaved to reveal blue and brightness. I sought solace by the pool at Anslow Park where house martins circled, mapping out a thousand roller-coasters. They opened up my mind and through the sound of the winded reeds I slowly settled, circled by the kestrel. Even the young plantation trees darkened the landscape as they grasped the land. Bright red berries clustered on the Guelder Rose, like spent gobstoppers, enlivening the landscape, as do holly berries in winter. The cooling towers stood, concrete-grey, like three doorways into the horizon, the scene of summer's exit to come.

The days remained static, like the pendulum paused at its zenith. A horizon of cloud lay across the tip of my slender tree and even the sunset was subdued, reduced to a line of peach below as the fixed sky hung. Foliage was paused, some oak leaves lay crisp, others hung amongst the green, their colour sucked out to an unfeasibly lifeless, institutional magnolia. The hollows were patient, their silence only punctured by the green woodpecker. Beech sprigs hovered, leaves outstretched, as if ready for a laying on of hands. The wooded air wrapped around; the spirit of the woods.

Two days later the spirit of the woods was in abundance as cool bright summer sun shone through the open canopy of pines at Blithfield. A return of summer, creating light and shade. The human eye can deal with brightness and shadow so much better than artificial means, and I took in the range of variously lit trunks diving into the deep fernery, splashing up shining foliage above. The ferns, still fresh, sat with fronds at oblique angles, greenfinches amongst them sounding shrill. This was what I needed. The deep field universe of ox-eye daises in the meadow was now an expanse of darkening matter, petals curled to grip fading yellow cores that were dry and disintegrated when touched. Butterflies, too quick for my eye, worked the remnants and it was still a glorious place to be. Over the stile, Stansley Wood is a darker, ancient, semi-natural woodland, where the ferns are restricted, as is the light. Here, the stripped oak rots from root to tip. Branches scatter the floor and its dark eyes look out over an oiled pit of a pond that slowly devours further snag trees; a lifeless hollow within the green. The head of a triceratops lies in the wood; a tree stump on its side that is given meaning automatically by my mind. Its snout sniffed the air as I passed, its knotted eye cast down. I left it to decay into the earth and be reunited with atoms of prehistory. Acorns, in their tight beanie-hat cups, sat ready to swell, surrounded by pitted leaves. There is growth in the woods yet. A picture-book goldfinch topped a thistle at the edge of the wood, as black crows complained above the heat-hazed corn, when suddenly the rotating calls of three oystercatchers took me back to the coast and the lazy summer weather of April. I returned through the heart of Needwood, pausing at the Meynell Ingram where I found a Stairway To Heaven, a bright corn-coloured ale with the aroma of summer. Sitting there in the sun, it became one of my all-time greatest pints, up there with Ram Tam, enjoyed by the sea at Port Logan, Fortyniner in October sunshine at Beer and another, whose name escapes me, on the bright shores of Loch Lochy.

The season had turned and I had to follow and having accepted the change of direction it was easier, if not exciting; although not for the dead shrew I found in the grasses at

Anslow Park, its beady eyes open, looking through the fine whiskers that circled its snout. It looked alive and inquisitive as it peered up from its final home, so much so that I expected it to run when I stroked its head. It was a smooth fragile being that gave a tingle of life to my fingertip. How we attach our values, and even personalities, to wildlife, from the adorable dormouse to the villainous magpie. As I moved on, a thrush preened on a solitary post, before a swallow approached, dipped steeply down to take something from the surface of the pond with an audible crisp splash, before leaving the scene.

The weather was set fair and back at the local ford the reflected willows rotated, unstable around their root, gyrating stalagmites in a flooded cave reaching upwards towards the light. The reflection made the shallows seem like a sky-deep pool, the vertical fronds of green enticing me in. Leon disturbed the surface with a stick and the illusion was broken into cubes by ripples intersecting with those deflected from the bank.

Elsewhere, deep in the undergrowth, below a sycamore, bramble leaves shone white, the sticky excretions on their leaves reflecting summer's light. Mixed in were leaves from beech to nettle, each using the light in their own way, producing every hue and shade of green, crossed by dark branchlets and filtered by diffuse seeded grasses before me. Later, as the sun descended out of sight I looked up at the birch leaves being picked out by the rays. Individual leaves went from a dry light olive to a deep green. The pattern on each was different, but all had their subtle V-shaped ridges and curves visible or accentuated to some degree. The patterns and shadows changed with the breeze, which was gently blowing the sun towards them, a solar wind. The fine twigs were divided along their length into light and dark, some catching the light boldly. The sun was attentive and almost seemed conscious of its life-giving power. As the horizon neared, the sun flickered too, interrupted by the top of a sole tree at first, before being fully tempered, apart from

94

the occasional diamond of light. All against a matt blue sky as a pigeon's curdled call skipped lazily through the cooling air.

Today queen ants began their nuptial flight. Against the setting sun they rose slowly and silently, like bright white confetti floating upwards, time reversed as the pendulum started to fall.

Against the midday sun at Brankley the teasels were edged bright as they rocked back and forth, feeding a host of insects. The cornflower had lost its brilliant hue as it radiated across the spectrum, saturation descending towards a heritage paint swatch. But there were plenty of tones to enjoy, from the scraggy mauve on the teasel, through raining purples to the vibrant dry yellow-gold alloy of the corn.

By the evening, rays of sun panned out to hold the cloud aloft, for these past few days had been summer-soft. Gentle warmth, evening cloud and subtle breeze. The goldfinches continued to call from their perch and a greenfinch underscored the day with a linear call. Once again there was a pink veil on the western horizon. The air was prominent, hanging still, cooling. Eventually the scaffolding of light gave way and the sun broke free, splitting the cloud and spilling out onto the lake to be reflected into the sky once more. Such is an ordinary summer's day. The hollows, bereft of birdsong and breeze, buzzed. There was a notable humming, an electric charge impeded by the leaves. In the hedgerow the snowberry provided a reminder of winter, its matt white berries sphered by subtle shadow, and its pink eggshell buds like miniature Easter decorations. A plant of the seasons.

The sun's rays were then thrust upward, fearing the roughness of the stubble in the field below. My mind was free once more, enjoying the expanse of the meadow, reclaimed and released from the darkness of the trees surrounding, moving on from the darkness of midsummer. And then the realisation came that I am not immune, I am also life and have silver in my stubble. I too am at midsummer, even though my consciousness seems to exist independent of time.

Just when I thought the evening had delivered more than I could bear, the sun reached the horizon and it was truly ablaze, an intense crater of molten light. But still the veil of pink remained, its subdued tone increasing the brilliance of the burning red sphere. Then it was gone and all that remained was a fire blanket of cloud.

IX

EXTRAORDINARY THINGS

4 August to 18 August

August came in as it should, sultry and tired. The decline of summer, trees sombre and a lack of spirit in nature, but soon the robin will begin its autumn song. I couldn't change the month, but I could view it from a different location and I was ready to extend my search, ready for new landscapes, ready to escape this pigeon-saturated, silted hollow for a short while. Hopefully to find extraordinary things on the Isle of Mull and in Northumberland, but that will come; for tonight I was at home. Here the clover was rising for its third cut, overcoming and feeding on the dense air. My slender tree was a silhouette cut precisely from a paper-bland sky. All the action was above, where the cloud rippled as if caught in a haze, and the sun lay in wait. The rooks' nests sat high, like benign parasitic growths amongst the green. The sun tried to lift the scene, but the humid air did not need its warmth. There was tension by the brook, splashing, rustling, squealing. A sparrowhawk was involved in some way or another, but I could see no more. I found another sparrowhawk, lying dead in the verge, bullet-shaped, with angelic white breast feathers belying its killer instinct. The young here had been lost to a magpie, and now an adult had been lost too.

After a few days the sultry conditions broke and we headed north through spray and under cloud to escape the darkness of midsummer in search of extraordinary things in the contrasting landscape of Scotland. There was mist hanging in the valleys and cloud smothered a ridge of trees as we emerged into an invasive drizzle at a nature reserve for lunch. I watched pond skaters, like swallows operating in two dimensions, before departing once more. The skies darkened, a wet concrete grey flooding down from the high land of the lakes, and we passed Heart Wood in Tebay Gorge. There was highland cloud, lower than the hills, reminiscent of that which had chased us down Gleann an Fhiodh a couple of years before.

We eventually arrived at Grey Mare's Tale, where the sky splits against the hill and the water falls. We had business unfinished here from a previous year. "It's quite amazing how the clouds reach the hills," said Isla. We pitted ourselves against the hill and rose steeply up a side of this classic glacial valley. Moffat Water had milled the valley floor flat and it shone metallic. The valley seemed to suck the sunlight towards us, and we watched as it descended the throat of the valley to be swallowed whole. Taken, like me, by the wild landscape, the rush of water, the visual avalanche as Loch Skeen opened out suddenly, the flatness contrasting markedly with the hills. A few steps further and there was peace as I stepped out of the wind. There was much to take in: reflected sky against dark hillside, lone trees on miniature islands. Static rocks, lively with mosses and grey and olive lichens, rippled within the swirling pool of mercury. The black of the mountain's shadow was broken by a calm white noise, a stream of data stored on the surface. But there was no code, no encryption: the message was clear. We set off on the steep descent back, scrubbed by the wild, the burn had erased the urban stains. The sun skated the heathers and Leon led the way, "une force tranquille". "Daddy, I'm following your footprints so I know where it's safe to go," said Isla.

Travelling through Glen Ogle the next day, the loch splintered the light which went on to sharply define the hills. Crisp in the light, cloud only touched the highest mountain. Forest floors were cast in light and shade and pine roots clawed the shallow-earthed crags. The wind carried us over to the Isle of Mull. A thin slice of cloud curved away over the Sound of Mull, which was silence. A pint of Monk of Iona was as smooth as the bay, but unfortunately more cloudy. The distant mass of Dun da Ghaoithe faded into the sky as bats painted rings of darkness. I was delivered.

The return to cooler conditions was like being taken back in time as I took in the fresher air and fresher greens on the short coastal walk to the lochan in Aros Park. Mossed trunks rose, green from within green. A black burn gravitated to the sea, through the pine needles that beaked the woodland floor, to jump the final steps, droplets leaping from the edge before rejoining the spout into the sea. I continued with a spring in my 200-pound step to a spot where water tumbled in, and trickled out, of a dark rust-based pool where the reflected ferns created an impression of a faded masterpiece of a romantic grotto. Further on I stopped at a pier looking back over the bay, the clear water revealing the beauty of ordinary things in the shallows of the sea. At the lochan even the pace of light seemed to have slowed as bright points advanced calmly towards me. It was a pleasant spot, but a single brilliant magenta rose with vivid yellow centre seemed more notable than the entire lochan.

Another day and at Glengorm, a tall larch stood dragged east by the winds, its trunk and broken barbed branches splattered with shaggy olive lichens. Nearby, several sycamores stood close, granite coloured trunks making them appear like lichen-covered stone forms. And further on nature's debris had been stood on end and arranged for unknown meaning. Standing stones, one of the few human constructions that add to the landscape. Simple, powerful, they seem to indicate connection rather than possession. Under distant skies we followed a causeway across a colourful marsh to a point where we were surrounded by upthrusts of rock, presumably volcanic in origin. We were in sight of Ardnamurchan and the saw-edged isles of Coll and Tiree. Amongst the rocks with white-grey lichens, one was splashed with gold and a lone haven for sea pinks. I found a cosy spot in the rocks, sheltered from the westerly wind and looking south. Plants grew here too, a sole, diminutive, flowering dandelion amongst them. Here I could hear the sea rather than the wind. Isla joined me, "Leon, do you want to come down here? It's really warm, cosy and echoey!" We then climbed the remains of the medieval fort Dun Ara and paused to view the truly bell-shaped blues of the harebell amongst the shallow mass of heather deep in colour. The flowers here seemed to be smaller, but perhaps more concentrated in colour. From the ruined fort the sky was a dark mirror of the Ardnamurchan peninsula and the Cuillin were faded fins on the horizon, breaking the surface of the sea and slashing the clouds. Martyn Bennett put this landscape to music in two eponymously named tunes that unfold to a view of the Cuillin shrouded in mist. My father had visited Skye with the Oread Mountaineering Club in July 1964 to traverse the Main Cuillin Ridge, a must for experienced rock-climbers. They camped in Glen Sligachan for access to Clach Glas and Blaven on the first fine day, before exploring a new route on Marsco Buttress and moving onto Gars-Bheinn and the Main Ridge. Skye and the Cuillin will be another trip for me.

We returned to Tobermory and eventually the darkness and rain crossed the water and arrived with us. The Sound of Mull changed from black to the silver of the sky as we were washed under grey. The soft cadence of summer rain filled the air before we set out again. Coig and Dervaig didn't capture us and we settled by the Mishnish, a body of water that seems to sit on, rather than in, the landscape. The sun was as watery as the boggy moor as we completed the short climb of the once volcanic vent of 'S Airde Beinn to circuit Crater Lake. It is a fine short walk through tussocks of fanned green grasses with banded yellow tips, heathers, wooded grey at the base and colour in the bogged earth from the lava-orange points of fire of a bloom unknown to me. Leon and Isla enjoyed the interactive deep soft mossy growths of green, yellow and red. There was little wildlife to be seen, just a froglet, black slugs and the telegraph-pole grey of the hooded crow. We descended out of the wind and I found the peace I found on our arrival in Mull, but had soon forgotten.

I have little interest in manmade forms that sit on the landscape but, as well as standing stones, I do enjoy sculpture in a natural setting, especially when it is formed from natural or recycled materials. So Calgary Art in Nature was a natural destination and one that affords a fine view of the silver of Calgary Bay between the basalt lava flows. The natural beauty, born of a violent volcanic origin still visible in the landscape, is built upon a foundation of ancient rock. The changes and violence continue in a subdued form, such as trees that succumb to the wind. "I love trees that have been pulled up. Look at all the roots," said Isla, continuing, "and then the tree lies down", as she passed the circle of root-filled earth, a sunken spoked wheel in the woods.

Calgary is extraordinary to human eyes; the shell-silver beach underlines a pure aqua. Tiny fragments of shells decorate the surface in shades of white, through silver-grey, to black. Beneath is a moon-grey sand. The tide came in slowly, spiralling currents navigating the ripples of the sand. The shallow wavelets of the incoming sea picked up the lightest black particles and cast them across the silver sand to settle in linear patterns and be recast. At the far end of the bay, fractured rocks had taken the sun's warmth and sat in the silver sand adorned by silver and yellow lichens. As we left a sudden shower came and stole the aqua blue. On our return we stopped at Loch Frisa, deep in the landscape and home of the extraordinary sea eagles of Mull. We sat for some time with no reward, other than the landscape itself.

Our good fortune with the weather continued for our fourth day on the island. It was how I remember the Highlands – the lengths of glistening water and the series of hills falling towards the lochs and fading in shades of blue-grey to those on the horizon. At Loch Ba the air was comfortably chilly and the sun strong, detailing the fine

101

arrays of the larch and reflecting off the wet rocks on the hillside. The weather and landscape reminded me of Glen Nevis, a place we had previously enjoyed in both sun and rain. Wisps of cloud teased the tops briefly, delivering the merest misting of water to us. The approach was pleasing, the loch small, with tree-topped promontories, and in proportion to the surrounding hills. The curves of the water's edge and forms of the trees and hillside engaged the eye; this may not be a wilderness, but nature is firmly in control. The many birch trees were stone-grey, with a story to tell, and every fingernail-sized leaf was scorched brown on the edge by the wind. But today it was still, lapping water could be heard and on the shore lay a lamb, plucked fleece surrounding a carcass picked clean. White-tailed sea eagles have been seen feeding on the shores near here. "That was amazing," said Isla after a buzzard-sized bird swooped before us and exited over the loch. In the last birches before the open head of the loch came a chattering of many finches, so busy as to make identification difficult, but Leon and I settled on there being dozens of joyous chaffinches, many in chasing pairs. I felt I had reached an equilibrium, swung back from the shock of connectedness, but this place was special.

I returned hand in hand with Isla and she asked why she shouldn't look at the sun. After explanation, the topics flowed fast and after dealing with what the Moon is made of, Isla asked, "You know the sky goes on and on and into space and further? How the world started is a really tricky question. We've got the world, but if we didn't have it, nothing would exist, so how did it start?" I was soon bogged down and reached the end of what I could comfortably explain, and then we couldn't recall how the conversation had started, but concluded it was probably a question about pebbles with holes in.

Later we drove along the shore of Loch na Keal, as I'd read it was a prime wildlife spot. We were looking for somewhere to stop and the first place had several people with binoculars and spotting scopes. They were set on a pair of sea eagles in a pine on a ridge above. We all got a view of the birds perched when suddenly the male flew over the loch, broad and commanding – with a menacing eye, according to Leon, who captured the event, if not the eye, in a drawing later. We rounded the spectacular coast, past basking seals on the Scarisdale rocks and on under the towering cliffs at Gribun to views out across Inch Kenneth to the lines of Staffa. A different side of Mull.

I awoke to another side of the weather and the other side of the bay was barely discernible through the rain and cloud. Half a dozen geese arose in a V shape from the mist up towards me, resolving from grey to black beating forms, rising through the all-encompassing wetness. The boats floated on what might have been the sky and the smell of the sea attached itself to the mist and was immersive. Veils of the vapour moved horizontally by. Later, the mist lifted and the trees became clouds, but it didn't last and the mists returned. The deep yellow ochre of the seaweed shone through as we returned to Loch Ba to sample it in the changed conditions. New streams had appeared, running across the grass that lay dragged down with the flow. The hills rose and faded to sky, sometimes appearing as shadow lands, like tears across the sky. Swollen burns stormed down the slopes, white through the gloom. "All my favourite walks have been in the rain," said Leon. The chaffinches met us at the shores of the Loch. They skipped over the tussocked grasses before flocking over our heads to the shelter of the birch, which now surrounded a perfect tumbling burn. "Wow!" said Leon as the birds went by. The loch faded to unknown lands and Isla saw the same. "Daddy, the loch looks like it fades into the sea," and it fooled the brain into thinking it was a great expanse. Swallows floated this deepened white to grey scene, rising and falling above and below the shaded horizon. Solitude's spirit resides in the mist here.

Leon and Isla were in their element, walking the streams, jumping puddles and being drenched. I felt the elements that had worked the birch, pushed by the wind and weighted by the rain. The loch had risen and waves lapped the skeletal lamb. Eventually the cloud lifted to reveal the lower green of the far shore, the tops still hidden as the cloud had only risen so far. The loch was now dark, the swallows no longer supernatural. Then the drizzle turned to driving rain and the wind became powerful. The loch was otherworldly once more and we got thoroughly soaked. That evening I retreated from the wet and overlooking the sculpted bay listened to the rain and *Diamond Mine*, a soundtrack of life in a Scottish coastal village, deeply satisfied and content.

"Feel this one, it's proper soft," said Isla as next morning we engaged with the young larch by Loch Torr. There was a large rowan in between. I'd seen few so far and this one had light bark patched by dark moss, supporting a scraggy top. The trees became an aside as a hawk flew up the path, directly above us, low and calling. Beneath us there were deer tracks on the path and onwards a swollen black burn, churned white and bridged by a fallen pine. It was edged by rowan, beech and a young birch that was more twig than leaf. We saw another hawk chased by crows and then a pair of red kites soaring for some time above the trees, the trailing edges of their wings noticeably ragged. We'd been richly rewarded, yet we'd only walked a couple of miles as we were keen to get to the pub, where my Scottish rarebit and Maverick ale was good.

We returned to Calgary Bay. Yesterday's rain had created a new stream across the sands. Its course was natural, free from human engineering and intervention. It emerged from the machair as a tight channel before it widened and curved through the sands, creating a curved canyon with steep sides and a flat bottom. The cliffs on the outside of the curves were constantly undercut by the turning stream, the tops occasionally giving way to disrupt the flow and be levelled onto the base of the stream. Opposite, the cliffs were left unaffected. The water then dispersed into a delta, rivulets carving a tree in the sand. The branches meandered down to the sea, carrying fragments of matter and rolling grains of sand; only to be wiped away by the reaching tide.

I traversed the beach where the sea meets the shore and saturates a band of sand dark and reflective. I cast my mind to the path at Dunstall where waves of grass broke into clover. The sea provided a crashing dynamic and all that was the same was the sound of the wind. It was time to leave this isle, and the places were linked in my mind at least. Given the power of the landscape here, the pleasure I had found in my ordinary surroundings at home seemed the more remarkable.

That evening there was a departing sky; smooth high peach coloured clouds leaving the hills alone as they headed for the mainland, resolving to grey as they went. Beneath the spillage of green, the bay was coursed by trails of calm leading to a darker Sound of Mull beyond. At least I had Northumbrian skies to look forward to.

The cloud clung to us as we left, low, reluctant, plugging the glens before they dissipated to rolling lowlands under a large fragmented sky. From west coast to east, from highlands to low, from Scotland to England, to the blue and straw-yellow expanses of Northumberland, lined by Morse code hedgerows. Fields dotted with crows as dark as the streak of Lindisfarne across the sea, which was weighted at one end by the castle notching the sky, its defined human lines somehow part of the landscape.

We spend time on the Northumberland coast each year, drawn back by the extensive sands and our base this year had views from Fallodon in the north-west to Dunstanburgh Castle in the south. The Farne Islands and Bamburgh Castle were visible ten miles distant. Close by, a large pond, cornfields and pasture. The benefit of knowing this area was that I didn't feel compelled to explore, could take in the view and have a more sedate search for ordinary things. That evening, at low tide, we walked the beach in fading light.

The wet sands sloped to the sea like a burnished shallow bowl of bronze. Dunstanburgh Castle and cliffs were grey in the spray against a dark, soft grey sky, the deep teal sea shocked by daubs of white. Twenty curlews flew above us towards the sea; and then more. A kestrel hovered the dunes, and we left.

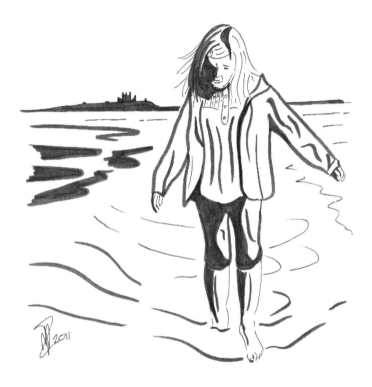

The sharpness of the rising sun was doubled by the sea. The mass of Dunstanburgh Castle looked paper-thin against the indistinct white band that formed the horizon. The grass in the field speckled bright and dark by light and shadow, whilst the pond reflected the trees on the far bank. Hedgerows railed inland, surrounding the cornfields. Pigeons and crows were immediately obvious as being busy, smaller birds flitted about, rabbits sat close to a magpie as a blackbird charged overhead. Swallows and martins cartwheeled over the pond, whilst swifts scythed above. Not to be outdone, two crows veered violently about, like electrons around an invisible core. Then hundreds of gulls, corvids and pigeons rose as a turmoiled cloud to scatter and resettle. A shower cloud passed from the west, rain shrouded the view, yet the sea and puddles reflected the sun.

This is a simple coast compared to the inlets and cliffs of Mull, and much of the Scottish west coast. A fair margin warmer too, as Leon and Isla got their time in the sea. The banked sand was patterned by every advance of the tide as the broken wave lost momentum, peaked and returned, leaving an outline reminiscent of last week's landscape. The bass swell and treble roll of the incoming tide provided a classic summer soundscape. Add in the visual expanse, the feel of the sand on bare feet, salt and seaweed in the air and it's the landscape at its most visceral. Yet a few yards back in the dunes it was quiet, grasses imitating the sea and a wild rose mounded amongst them. Like Mull there were harebells, but also purple bloody cranesbill.

Later, hundreds of jackdaws passed over from the fields, and the reflections of the trees by the pond were drawn long as the sun began its setting. The cloud was a constant height, shrinking away in bands of white to blue-grey, the sun bright to the west. I yearned to be up the coast at Bamburgh, where the evening sun shines along the beach, doubling and retouching the light to spectacular effect, although capturing this event on camera has possessed my evenings too often in previous years when based there. Just as enjoyment can be spoilt by feeling the need to understand, pleasure can be reduced by trying to commit nature to film. And then the feeling grew as light was cast across the landscape towards the sea, like a river of bright wine, splashing the castle into brightness against the dark sky. The sky was clearing from the west and the scene was set, but I was far from the stage. I could picture the events at Bamburgh in my mind's eye: forget the bulk of the castle, it is the sunsets reflecting off the wet rippled sand and shallow pools that dominate. The carefree walks that go on and on, to Greenhill Rocks or beyond and the return to Stag Rock where the final sinking of the sun can be seen. The edge of the world, where landscape meets a fiery end. Thankfully, for my peace of mind at least, the colours were tempered by a band of cloud on the horizon and I could rest. The search for ordinary things can become engrossing.

As darkness fell the ducks gathered and called along with other birds in the hedgerows. Some high clouds were stained red and from the cloud a full moon appeared over my shoulder, to the east over the castle, like a pearl emerging from within a shell. Like the sun it reflects, it defined the edges of the cloud, but its action was limited to a circle perhaps three times its diameter, more as day light faded. The dark trees merged with their reflection in the pond and the still of night was upon us. The moon silvered the cloud fully and the alarm call of the blackbird came to close the evening and turn the day over to night. In the half-light wing-beats could be heard and the moon was a joy through a lens.

Having walked the dunes in the morning we sat outside the Ship Inn, with brewing in progress. The Ship Hop ale had travelled the five yards well. Leon and I watched the swallows over the green and there were plenty of perky sparrows about. They always are here on the coast, but rarely seen at home. Fallodon is a couple of miles away and Viscount Grey of Fallodon wasn't keen on the bird, writing in 1927, of an unattractive bird, with an offensive chirp, untidy nests and having the "manner of thieves". Strange how the book is titled *The Charm of Birds*. Richard Jefferies, in his 1880s book *The Open Air*, noted the sparrow was often despised, but like me, he saw the "most animated, clever little creatures".

Walking back along the beach, dunlin scampered the boundary of the sea as the shorn rock-edged mass of Castle Point seemed to float improbably on a film of water which stretched across the bay. Whilst the sun brightened the breaking waves, greying cloud gathered to the north, showering the sea the same colour, losing the horizon. A pair of terns headed south, heads dipped towards the sea, occasionally lifting to look forward, pausing to hover when sustained attention was required. A dead seal lay on the beach, mouth agape, teeth biting the air.

At the end of the bay there are large stones that have sunk into the sand, polished and black. The disturbed currents divot the sand to create moats of clear water around them. Where these rocks become more numerous several juvenile pied wagtails gathered and one pair chased and battled furiously, knowing each other's every turn, translucent wings lit by the low sun. As I turned back so did the terns, lit against the slate sky as sharply as their wings are shaped, darting over the sea in search of food. The tide had turned and the beach was wiped clean reflecting the colours of the sky.

The next morning brightness and landscape were constant. Ducks glided on the pond, foliage nodded in the breeze and there was little to stimulate my mind. The gulls in the field rose, spiralling loosely as flotsam lifted into a whirlwind. They rotated clockwise and formed a tighter column that rose higher and higher until they seemed to meet the base of the cloud. Some gulls returned to the field, but others remained aloft as the column drifted southwards. Swallows dipped the pond, rings of light catching water visible from my distant vantage point. It was a restful scene, but I didn't want to rest. At least by the coast the waves are constant. I walked through the ridge and furrow of the beach at low tide, to the expanse of smooth, the sun reflecting intensely all the while. The flatness and extensiveness seemed to unfold and free the last corners of my mind, opening it up, an inverse origami, making simplicity, removing complexity, leaving the mind free to find its own form.

The low tide revealed the field of giant pebbles, dried to grey, busy with birds including a pair of fighting young wagtails, still locked in synchronous flight, white wing bars whirring. At the base of the castle, the ruins of man's attempt to posses the landscape, clumps of grass broke the surface of the mere; from many around the edges to few within the centre. I watched the fulmars soar over the basalt cliffs, grey columns stained olive, white and black; vertical on a horizontal strata base. The flat sea took on the colour of the sky from horizon to shore, a spectrum from metallic grey, through white, to the deep blue of a child's painting – and how I wish I could paint like a child.

That evening there was golden light and I felt drawn to Bamburgh once more, where the tide was more restful, taking a slower, deeper breath. Each wave slowly advanced up the shore without a notable crash, rather a gentle crescendo, and then an extended fade: the pendulum of the tide. Add to this the ability to walk the shore for several miles, with the nearest other person a mere speck on the horizon, and you have found the essence of ordinary things. Here you can literally retrace one's steps and see human impact on the landscape washed clean.

Isla picked up a feather and scribed its point across the back of my hand before saying, "I'm your proper daughter now. I signed my name on you. I signed my name on you!" And then, "I really like walking on this beach in the evening." There were a few dozen swallows low above the beach; unusually, many landed and pecked at the sand. With the sun on my back I followed my shadow to an anthropometrically perfect stone on Islestone Rocks where last year I'd watched gannets bomb the water. This year it was Arctic tern.

The oblique light picked out the recordings of the outward tide in the sand, but the sunset was barred by thick cloud, edged by fire with an icing of white above, all reflected by foil sands. I waited, watching the castles in the clouds, as light is quick to exploit and wrong step any weakness. Slowly the sun sank to the base of the barring cloud and a furnace of light burned through, radiating beams from its core, trimming the deep purple cloud orange. It soon faded though and the sand turned a shade of grey, but simultaneously the moon rolled onto the horizon opposite, sitting calmly and warmly tinted. To the south of this east–west balance of celestial bodies, spectral clouds leapt from the dusky sky, which suddenly took on the red of the sunken sun, like the breath of a dragon at rest.

The next day was dense and watery as we headed across the purple heather moors. The mist was flat and, at lower levels, hanging in the trees. There was heavy rain, and toads, toadstools and other fungi amongst the heather, birch and granite. It passed and the sun brought a remarkable spring freshness and life to the green. And then, standing by a still lake, I was transported across the seasons once more. Yellow birch leaves on the wind with the swallows, eventually falling to float on the reflected sky. Those near my feet were wet and bright against dark mossy grass and the granite. The giving birch were old, trunks grey and hidden by olive lichens. The characteristic peeling bark only appearing higher up amongst the branches. Over Corby's Crags a broad low rainbow traced the edges of a heather-dressed ridge so that the purple heather merged with it and seamed into the sky through a spectrum of colours.

On our return structured clouds, with heavy sea-coloured bases, supported towers of billowing white that hung above the water, still, in a baby blue sky. Horizon clouds built distant isles as sparrows fed at my feet. An hour after sunset the western sky was a light blue, clouds black and fearful. Opposite, a night blue with smooth-blown clouds teased the waning moon, with its edge of darkness casting silver over the sea.

Early the next day a sparrowhawk spooked swallows low over the dunes, which hid the flat sands beyond. The stream running onto the beach was dynamic, reflecting rivulets of light willowing out towards the sea. Each wavelet and ripple cast shadows and focussed light onto the surface below, and in turn to my eyes. Hollows and rises built under the main flow until the wave stalled and then broke in series up-stream, before returning to its calm undulating flow. Limpet shells were dragged along the sand, smoothly at the margins or taking ridges and furrows at speed. The shrill terns and distant waves of low tide completed this wonderful ordinary scene.

Down the coast, before Cullernose Point, the land slips meekly into the sea, which rolled gently onto the rocks where the oystercatchers called. The land and sea at equilibrium, balanced and comfortable with their position. At Cullernose Point the masses of land and sea do battle. Lines sharply drawn, rock overhangs the sea, which tries to undermine the cliffs that fall defeated, to be rounded in pieces on the shore, the gorse above providing a futile second line of defence. We rested on the shore, the sun reddening my eyelids and the sea rippling the air which carried the gentle energy to my ears. The elements transferred to my mind. Jet-streams of cirrus spoked the sky, converging at a point somewhere over the ocean. The dry barnacled rock was tufted with crisp seaweeds. The strata roll like whale-backs to the sea, which gulped greedily as it looked to consume the shore and rescue the life held in the pools above. Isla prodded the various creatures in them. "If you poke them with a bit of seaweed they squirt at you! There's a baby lobster!" Leon watched the seaweed in the waves and Isla allowed a ladybird to explore her hands. Then they lay on rocks, arms outstretched into the oncoming tide. Behind the rocks, the water seeped gently into an inlet and its inexorable rise could just be gauged as it crept over the contours and barnacles. Time is visible here. I stood on the top of the largest whale-back, surrounded by clear blue water, and let time pass. When the tide reached the rounded boulders it dressed them in finest jet and they shone next to their drab neighbours whose time was yet to come.

As night fell, the sea matched the colour of the sky so that the horizon disappeared, only to be revealed by the rising moon, its peached orange face crossed by thin fingers of cloud. The raucous geese gathering on the mere fell silent, curlew gave a brief melancholy call and a little owl closed the day.

A final day in our summer haven and the polished wet beach of low tide was large enough to reflect the blue of the sky; it seemed as if we were walking in mid-air, accompanied by a brush-stroked reflection, floating out to sea to flounder on Jenny Bells Stone and come to rest on drawn sand, where water had sprung to map out a forest of trees, or a burial of roots. Further on these forms resembled flames imprinted into the surface, rising up the beach, reflections white-hot. A storm of jackdaws took flight beyond and circulated like flakes of ash, carried on the wind to settle amongst the corn.

When the tide turned, rolls of liquid glass slid along the level plain of sand, each one exploring new contours, adjusting and transforming the landscape before my eyes. The sound of breaking waves was constant. I stood in the shallows, amongst a matrix of brightness as the waves flowed by, my mind telling me I was travelling without moving. Then I was in the Dales, immersed in the sound of the falls; in the meadows with lapwing and curlew; walking the long grasses and clover. I was at home.

X

THE DOVE

20 August to 24 September

And then I was standing in a field like scorched sand, faded blades blunt in the dust. Many trees had dry-edged leaves, some yellow sprigs, even shots of red in the hedgerows, like rust on a beached hull. Rose hips had a hue of the setting Bamburgh sun, neighbouring young rowan bent over, heavy-laden. Plantation trees stood green amongst the pale and fallen grasses, like Martians lost amongst flotsam on the shore. Their colour will soon be alien when they stand skeletal amongst the green. The cow parsley at Dunstall that reached for my eyes was stark and stiff, seed-heads like a collection of rolled oats. Blackberries gathered black and the acorns were plump. The lime had splashes of yellow, whereas the hawthorn had a more even fade and its crimson berries hung for harvest. The sycamore leaves were scruffy, spotted black and would be better fallen to the ground. Yet the patient ash was youthful, glorious and permeated by light. Parts of the woodland floor were spent and the herbage of the plantation lay without direction, ill-defined and crazed. Looking out from the higher ground the subtle changes in the trees were hardly apparent: their dominant green darkness surrounded and balanced the parched pasture whilst swallows fed above them. My rolling tide of grass and clover lay like a bank of stranded seaweed. The thistles were dressed by what might be fleece carried on the wind. Without me the pendulum had moved on. Two crows paused on the stiff breeze as they looked to carry the season: one last push will see it fall. And robins sang in the

115

hollow of the evening, filling the void, evacuating summer; like me, the season seemed ready to move on.

Primed, I noticed the robins each day and one evening there was robin song all around. I followed the sound of one and, finding its perch, I stood and watched as it sang a few yards away. It was half-lit by the sun as it paused to listen to another, or consider its next phrase, head at an angle, notes both rapid and drawn. I walked until I could hear them no more, until the dusty track turned to stone and the sun hurt my eyes. I cast them back to look over the fields. The rain had tried, but the air still tasted of dust as a young chiff-chaff repeated, looking for an answer amongst the hedgerow and yellowed bindweed. I was looking too, but not sure what for. The Dove Valley stretched out and I thought back to where I had started, understanding the landscape, listening to the nature around me, being moved. I wasn't sure if I'd swung back from it, or I'd caught hold, but I figured I was happy and carried on, returning to where the robin still sang.

Static, there was no need to move to be impressed; the rain came, slowly building until the sun joined and bright rainbows doubled. The up-shining sun lit the grey clouds yellow as they drifted away, dragging a streaked trail behind, patterned with yellow wisps. Against the firm sky blue, the clouds in the distance looked painted flat, yet bold in colour, and the warm light gave the landscape both richness and depth, getting under the canopy to reveal the secrets of the woods. The sky was drawn south to north, a tunnel rather than half sphere. I followed to higher ground where once more the robin approved, and the sky was of awesome magnitude and scale.

The bridleway at Dunstall was now dotted with leaves and the hedgerows were patterned with yet more new hues. We set out in sunshine, but within minutes there was rain. We sheltered under an oak, the clusters of leaves above us, dark against the sky. A sparrowhawk landed high in a nearby pine and called all the time we waited for the shower to pass. Leon kept watch. "I love looking at that tree," said Isla, pointing at a neighbouring tall pine, "You can see all of it from bottom to top." Isla went on to describe where the lambs had played between the limes, hiding in a hollow trunk, as we looked out over the site of the pigeon kills. I was excited by the prospect of the return of the mystery hawk, which perhaps overwinters here.

After the shower, the sun came bright and bejewelled the ash. Rowan-berry bunches were cast in light and shadow as we were surrounded by an amphitheatre of giant white mounded clouds. "It's nice, the rain is glinting off the plants!" said Leon. Once amongst them, the ash were yellowing, backlit by the sun into the fresh patterns of spring. An electric buzz of grasshoppers added to the atmosphere.

The twelve chimes of noon cut through the woods like the shafts of sunlight. The paths were greasy from the rain, another reminder of past and future, the cycle and turning of the year. Leon landed from a stile like a sack of potatoes. "I'm not particularly good at landings," he commented. The darkest of clouds loomed as we emerged from the wood. We moved quickly as the next cover was some way off. The thistles had lost their fleece and the rain came. We sheltered where the fox cubs had played. Beneath a maple and with the hawthorn, a ladybird appeared dull amongst the bright crimson berries. Leon and Isla went into the dark of the wood to shelter. I too ventured in as the rain became torrential. The wood was dark, sunbeams gone. The only brightness was from the raindrops making it through the trees and dropping from the leaves, as they gathered the light and carried it to the ground, where it sparkled amongst the

117

leaf litter. In the other direction the rain was invisible, only apparent through occasional touched leaves, as they weren't between the sun and me. When I reached Leon and Isla they'd been out the other side of the wood, feasting on blackberries, the evidence found across their faces. "They were very, very nice and had a sweet taste to them," said Isla. Still raining, we waited once more. Forced to pause, I sank into the leaf mould and mosses, immersed in the waves of rainfall, protected by the tree that stood with me. As it slowed we walked in the rain, led by my shadow, sun on my back, glistened clover on my sole. Looking back, the birch shone, as if bedecked by lights, bright enough to shine under the midday sun. Isla picked and ate a small red apple to add to her foraged brunch. As we went on the Trent Valley opened out, now filled by the showers. Water evaporated from the fields in wisps and whirlwinds, seemingly swept up by the swallows.

In the morning the raindrops on the lake were as bright and as dispersed as the yellow birch leaves on the land. By the afternoon the wind tested the drying leaves on the trees, but they held on and the air was clear, free of debris floating on the wind, free to hold the birds aloft, free to split and move the clouds and carry the closing August rays to earth, free to wrap around me, free now as the weaker leaves had already fallen, sprigs of oak and curlew beak pine needles amongst them. Soon the wind will be busy, stripping the hollows, filling the air, covering the earth, closing the season.

The hollows roared in protest, standing firm. The wind whispered as it left, giving no clue as to when it would return. The clover in the meadow nodded approvingly at its plans, the thistledown carried above by its friend. Higher still, a kestrel hung in the air as swallows and martins swarmed. I watched them slice over the cornfield, making patterns as complex as the clouds floating behind. Then they rose against the blue, swirling above me like the leaves that will soon be carried on the wind. I left reluctantly, heading straight for their centre where they carried on oblivious, for they have a longer journey ahead of them. I paused where my shadow had been cast long by golden light seven months before to take on another offering of nature's glory. Perhaps August isn't so bad after all.

As I tramped back home, someone in a Lamborghini revved past me and then returned, stopping deliberately near me, before speeding off once more. I looked to the hedgerow; if someone finds as much pleasure in an acorn as others find in a luxury car, imagine how rich their world is.

We saw August out at Blithfield, where we walked the golden splashes that decorated the paths and shrubs. The ferns were turning; purple loosestrife was weighed down and contorted. I stood under the sycamore that had provided the first fresh canopy of the year in late March. The leaves were now in a tired and pitted state. A bee had its head plunged deep into a blackberry flower, extracting the remnants of summer.

September, and it was more like summer than it had been for quite some time. At Anslow Park dragonflies were locked in pairs, birds and grasshoppers called, and the trees rustled dryly. Red berries shone, like the guts of the season ripped out and laid out for the birds to feed on; leaves, the colour of dried blood, surrounding. All below a high patchwork of white and blue, escaped from a celestial line and blanketing summer in a vain attempt to protect it, keep and preserve. But there were no swallows and martins skimming the shallow and reduced pool. It was like looking back on an incomplete memory of summer. The thick air and warmth browning my skin will depart; time says so. My search for ordinary things will soon end and I shall have to provide my own warmth. Like a flake of summer, a small lilac butterfly scattered along between the trees as the thistledown floated calmly, looping with the gusting breeze. It was a particularly beautiful day. Even the blackthorn sloes, coated matt, couldn't resist giving away their spheres and reflecting the point of light that is our sun. Change brings new ordinary things, but I will miss those that have become extraordinary to me.

ψ

Since my last visit to Dunstall the lime had been hit broadside by autumn, with golden shrapnel cast about. Amongst the gold, pigeon feathers were dispersed and we carried on towards a buzzard call. "I've got that sparrowhawk call echoing in my head," said Leon as a strange cry, like an anguished duck, came from the trees. Our approach flushed the buzzard and it circled and called, impressive in size, as we stood beneath the mighty beech, its canopy with a multitude of branches and countless leaves, like a new sky over this calm corner with views to the north. "This is my favourite bit of Dunstall," said Leon, and then looking up, "If I could just sit on top of that tree. Or fly." We discussed the goshawk, that it may have been a juvenile passing through looking for its own territory. Unrestricted by roads and boundaries, it could have spent the summer nearby or further afield. We shall never know.

Later, I set out to explore paths I had ignored by the River Dove at Marston. It was black, barely showing the towed weed as silver-knifed willow leaves were drawn by the breeze. A heron lifted as a lone cormorant perched on a snag tree. All the time the church bells pealed.

I returned the next day to explore the Dove upstream and I wondered why rivers bring calm. Cradled by the landscape it is channelled and delivered, like the finch flying with the wind. Rivers carry the spirit of the uplands across the landscape, washed down liquid, below gas and through solid earth, captured by the landscape in the oxbow. In return the river captures the sky by reflection. And the sky captures us all.

Amongst the steady drizzle I progressed along the bank towards the birdsong and emerged into a new landscape along a path I'd not taken before. I felt joy at being able to connect to the river. In the meadow there was a new green, with a hint of blue. There were willow, alder, hawthorn and mature ash; the largest filled the sky with the form of a thunder cloud. Close by elderberries hung black on red veins. I wished I'd taken this path before, but that would have denied today's discovery. The quiet was such that I could hear the return of leaping fish. As the water flowed by, the reflections of the ash, reeds and willows remained still. Almost perfect representations, only disturbed by the occasional fish as the drizzle was too fine to disturb the surface. Further upstream the water ran in calm rapids, producing countless individual sounds as it rounded a sandbank, like audible leaves on a tree. I returned to realise I had left the birdsong around the giant ash, which the robins were attempting to describe.

Another day, and I had to see the river again. It only roars where there is a weir. The landscape is only sharp where there are buildings. The sky is only straightened by the contrail. Few places are truly ordinary, apart from the wildlife within. Here it is the swan, the moorhen and pied wagtail. And then, as it started to rain, I stood looking downstream and a kingfisher zipped the centre of the river, above the rings of water, low into the distance until even its special brightness could no longer be seen

At dusk, drawn once more, I took Leon to the river. "I prefer rivers with a bit of sound," he said as we pushed through the strong wind and coming rain. "I'm ready for some windy, and some rainy weather," he continued as close by an ash tree offered its leaves to the Dove. Then an unearthly haunting sound came from the half-light as two swans emerged in flight from that middle place. Straight and determined, their spectral white shaded to reveal their form against the grey, power belying their grace, beneath the new supernova in the plough.

We returned for a fifth day, with the full moon we'd last seen in Northumberland. The evening was still and clear, bar the dusk. We passed the home of the heron and circuited the oxbow in the dark, becoming more fully aware of the sounds painting the landscape in the absence of light.

I wasn't going to visit again, but Leon was keen. Seven ducks sat on a stranded log in the oxbow, and a heron floated off above the water that was clear to blackness. The swans showed their grace, their feathers bright in the sunlight, fluttering in the breeze as if they could never support flight. The wind was thick, warm and firm, asking the willows to lie down and cross the river to join the swans reflected. The broad contorted willows refused, their decrepit trunks still able to support healthy foliage. Thirty to forty jackdaws lifted from the stubble, scattering blackness amongst the deepening cloud. The wind was due to bring rain. Like the cormorant, we just wanted to sit alone by the river, on the remains of the quarter-mile bridge. We imagined the steam train cutting through the flood plain on the embankment here, many faces looking out, the landscape consumed by eyes and now living in the memories of the few. Returning, Leon explored the pillbox, put there to defend the landscape from invaders. I stopped once more and, sitting on a fence, took time to be on the flat plain. I realised that during these six days by the Dove I had not paused. I thought I could attend to detail on the move and that my eight months of searching meant I could connect to nature in an instant, with a capacity for a bandwidth that floods the mind. That was not the case.

Large clumps of dried thistles rattled in the wind as it forced the oxbow to flow once more, its clear waters lit where the ripples delivered the sunlight. Leon and I watched water skaters glide between the water lilies, their reflective bodies creating points of light spiralling above the weed clear below. "They're like water dodgems," said Leon, and their light was like an electric spark in a fairground's night. Dragonflies coursed above and yellow willow leaves were freed to the surface. The sky eventually cleared to lines of high cloud, mirrored in the tracks through the stubble below. The jackdaws appeared en masse, as bright as black can be.

At rookery wood the swallows had gone, but the rooks had returned to their nests atop the ash, circling in the air like spinning plates on sticks. The remnants of Hurricane Irene had crossed the Atlantic and created a circus in the trees, but they were not in a giving mood as they stood, leaves attached.

The following day and perhaps my last evening visit to Dunstall, for the full tour at least. I was enthused by the opportunity, keen to make the most of it in gales and the setting sun. The wonderfully black rooks delighted too, racing with the wind as they headed for the beamed sun. And back. And forth. And back once more. Leon and I were in our element, up the bridleway, sparrowhawk calling as before. Twelve foot of sycamore lay before us, near the turn-off for the mighty beech, which Leon wanted to visit. Our arrival prompted a single-file stampede of sheep; a hundred or so passed in a line from one hundred yards away. We passed many tan mushrooms, fungal in the grass, as we progressed to the limes with noticeably fewer leaves, many lying dry below. There was a low distant rumble of the gale, a soundtrack that seemed to make the loss easier. The young ash in the plantation were yellow, dynamic in the wind. The young saplings still reached up, some bare, just a slim finger of wood. Corvid cries came from the dark wood in motion. It was an exciting scene. In the mature woodland, trees lay uprooted, leaves and twigs littering the floor, and others made sounds as they fell. A tawny owl repeated, a violent close of a day. A close of a season.

The setting sun cast the landscape in the colour of the ash, as if it was seeping out of their leaves. The moon watched over us as we navigated the fading light, guided by a busy bat. The wind was fading too, but I could still sense recharging energy. The pond reflected the last of the light,

123

revealing the ducks in silhouette, as the moon played with the shapes in the clouds.

The setting sun was now a companion as my search for ordinary things was forced into shorter days. Once more it was the backdrop as, against it, the top of my slender tree rode the skyline like a matchstick at ignition. I was walking the twilight once more. The circuit of the Earth forced winter's evening options onto me, keeping me close to home, increasing the value of the light. The situation reminded me of the start of my search; then it was also a search for light, making full use of the day and exploring small pockets of time. Time and light, the macro ordinary. I had been attentive to the micro, but once more I was aware of the whole, like the layers of a bulb that all contribute to the bloom, when the time is right. I was so connected to this cycle that I felt compelled to withdraw and close my search, to fit in with the closing of the summer and drawing in of the probing light. It seemed disrespectful to ask anything of nature when it was time to rest.

The scent of autumn arrived, the coolness of air on my skin after a day of sun, which was setting as I stood in the dark of the rookery wood. Moving out, there was light over the fields, an orange horizon with purple wisps.

Leon described the sky as a tidal wave, with clouds breaking over each other, and we set off to Drakelow in an unlikely search for a terrapin. Isla's homework had a terrapin theme and I'd seen reference to a terrapin sunning itself here. We were welcomed by a large dark buzzard, as I have been welcomed before, wings outstretched and steady, primary feathers distinct. Dunnock song, treecreeper and crows crossed as I was webbed by a spider's thread. I felt lagooned in the crisp combination of breeze and sunlight as I looked out on a dried-up pool, surrounded by reeds dragged by the breeze, cracked silt dotted by pebbles; their bases wet stained, tops dried matt. A corner of grey cloud was teased from the greater mass like a tuft of fleece. It stained the fresh blue and morphed as we approached to sit and look over the water. Shortly, there were three heavy splashes, like large stones hitting the water, and a few yards before us a terrapin leapt and crashed through the surface. If Isla hadn't been engaged by blackberries, she would have seen it. Then an ancient heron circled the lagoon, which reflected in the sunshine, whilst below the grey of the rain. A swan with highlighted lines passed, landing as its reflection rose from the surface. The cormorants were gone, their stained haunts bare. Nearby a beech was open, branches revealed, its remaining yellow leaves bronzed and next year's buds apparent. It offered scant protection from the coming rain as I considered the neighbouring beech, which was greener, its branches less upright, more irregular, less compelling. I moved on into the rain, keeping close to the hedgerow that showered berries.

The following day at Brankley, the birdsong was as crisp as the autumn air. The freshness cooled my fingers. Finches led through hedgerows splashed with warm tones. With the cooling of the air comes the warming of the colours: greens ignite and warm the soul. The green woodpecker was where it had been before, calling from its hedgerow, visually salient on a protruding snag tree. Equally still, the young birch close by was sharing its green. Beyond, an oak had split, a third of its mass descended. Lines in an arched scar rose from the base of the trunk, eight feet high and three wide. Above the ancient wood pasture, two crows lazed in the breeze and rolled the gentle hills of the next valley. This is a place I struggle to leave. It always reflects the seasons with intensity. From bitter cold to in leaf, from bluebells through to the green darkness, and now the coming chill of autumn. I looked forward to the clasping mists of winter.

The next time I left home to continue my search, dark clouds were close. The trees were deflated to the grey of the sky before they succumbed to the mist of slashing torrential rain and they sat indeterminate and faded, layering up the valley side until they were cloud too. My slender tree extinguished, I stood looking at the ganzfeld sky and with the pink noise of rain my mind was free to see. And it did see. It saw the joy within me, to be within nature's storm. Later, after the rain had cleared the sun fired the trees to charcoal-black and they stood bold, greyness washed, their tops holding a sheet of purple cloud aloft so that the glow of the furnace was revealed, until they splintered and their darkness filled the sky.

Two evenings later the river was the sky, as grounded we ventured upstream. Blinds of Venetian cloud stratified the sun as six swans lined the Dove. A further two swans stood in the rapids, which played with the revealed rays. We stood by the mercury surface, with the rippled water sounding out the reflections. The far bank was vertical, cracked and holed, the near bank descended gradually in the green. Having navigated the pebble islands, Leon was reflected to darkness. Isla followed. "My favourite part of this whole river is this bit," she said. And it was a good choice. It was a cool and still evening that carried sound, and the heron, over a pair of snag trees that provide a perch to view the flood plain. We followed a single swan feather downstream, contrasted against the water, now dark. Nearby fish jumped, bright, silver, at times in threes.

The following day was a September day that could not be ignored, sunshine blue, and amongst the big trees my breathing slowed to contentment. Jackdaws clacked beneath specks of rooks before an evacuation of pigeons left the cover of the woods. I found myself reflecting on the year, focussing on and waiting for the colour. Summer wasn't falling today, just one leaf that spun calmly and dropped slowly. Furred spires exploded from the undergrowth of brambles and nettles, causing me to pause. Beyond the

126

yellow birch a dragonfly, a bright segmented abdomen in a cloud of wings.

I was keen to make the most of the dry ground and sunlight, so set out once more the next morning to Dunstall. The cry of a buzzard kick-started my connection at the point where I found intense affect in May. I took in the yellowing plantation oak, bright-edged by the sun. Teasel seed-heads dotted the dried grasses; blackberries held red as jettisoned leaves increased their covering of the bridleway. The shorn sapling ash lined up against their established neighbours, curling or grasping onto a fading singed yellow. A faded, scorched picture of spring. A fallen photograph splashed by autumn hues.

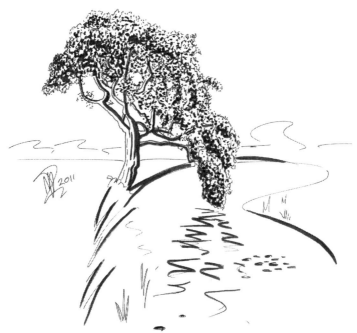

At dusk the Dove carried the reflection of the swans with ease and willows sat still on the edge, grained like photographic film, under a yellow filtered sky. Their focus was indistinct, trunks and supporting branches not apparent.

Moorhens split and dived within, running the water as they crossed the river, which was doing what it could to create a Bamburgh sky, doubling the glowing clouds. I trudged the flat brown tilled earth to the open oxbow where silver dried superstructures lined the bank and lily pads broke the reflected sky. I paused by a leaning alder that nearly touches the water, a painter's tree, forever frozen as it reaches for its reflection, attempting to cast an eye on its own form, forever denied. A painter's tree as I had seen its form before in a host of romantic landscape oils. Rays from the hidden sun were cast upwards from the horizon, like the beams from a vehicle approaching the brow of a hill, but I knew the sun would not appear again, not today.

XI

THE STEALING

26 September to 6th November

Equinox gone, the light evenings were retreating at the double. As nature cloaked the ordinary things ever earlier, I was resigned to no more evening searches at Dunstall. I was occupying the other place between night and day, between now and then, between bare attention and disregard. The sun lit the sky so that the land was captured under a falling golden leaf on a celestial scale. The restricted spectrum of light was only interested in picking out the reds and golds around me. Two geese passed and robins provided audio fireworks in the dusk, lighting up the cool evening air with patterns of sound. I rose into the cooling air, washed.

The cool evening air did not last and ordinary things were found in extraordinary warmth, as hot as midsummer. In the hollows the birds called, but were elusive, unlike the acorns that fell about us with surprisingly loud dull thuds on the dusty earth. They rolled to sit amidst the tired soil, baked satin shells lightly barred with dark lines grasping towards the tip from the light base. Isla picked one up. "Why are acorns so smooth and nice? Feel it!" she said. A squirrel shot by. "I saw its eyes and its tail and its mouth open. They're very fast," said Isla. "Where's it gone?" she continued, looking up at the oak. "There it is, right up there! It's gone so far, then it stretched itself and went up more," – she paused briefly – "come on then!" she ended before moving on to examine the acorn. "Wow!" she exclaimed as she opened it up, taking away the outer shell to reveal the seed, before continuing, "And that's where they sleep."

Later, the last gasp afterburn of summer had singed the leaves dry and produced an exhaust-blue sky. The shadows of the oxbow willows were cast far over the flat fields, reaching for their river beyond. A willow near the painter's alder was touched with luminous gold and the reflection allowed me to look down, yet up through its glory. From within came the sweet burbling song of the dunnock. As I moved on the heron was patient on a snag branch of the alder. It was reflected too, but it is of a form that cannot be enhanced, nor does it need balance. I reached the quarter-mile bridge and the low sun beamed across the flood plain, perpendicular, inspecting the land and highlighting every imperfection, lighting the weeds in the pasture golden. The light was washing the landscape to an entire autumn as I sat and enjoyed the calmest of golden moments my search could bring. Still elusive, several birds left me guessing as I let nature unfold before me. The sun lowered and melted away, the golden flow that had coated all around me was gone. Cool air filled the void and the landscape was reduced to itself. Returning, the willow had had its lustre taken, but the painter's alder remained a compelling form. And then the journeys began: an arrowhead of geese heading north, the sixty rooks heading east for their evening roost, and a pre-migratory flock of a few hundred house martins arrived, high, like a hole in the waning blue, testing my eyes, merging with the detritus within as a lone swan arced below.

October, and I shot to the heart of Needwood. Past perched hawk, coursing a blood flow of trees to Brankley where cool morning air and hazed light touched the grass-tipping dew. My search for ordinary things had missed two hundred ordinary dawns, but I am a night owl. As I approached them from the haze, there was clarity in the trees. The deep greens were relieved by fading oaks, spotted by berries, jewelled by yellow birch leaves and tired at the edges with blighted chestnut. Inside, the wood was full of light, unusually expansive, calm with beech yellowing from branch tips towards their heart. The ancient leaning oak sat in its own beam of light, having seen one hundred thousand dawns, or double. I peered into the crevices of its tortured bark, black amongst the rutted and twisted olive plough lines, its surface spotted by occasional dried birch leaves. On its dark side there was less deep shadow, but also a gaping hole through to the light. But this oak still gives, and its acorns landed at my feet. I moved on, sat amongst the corvid cries, and took in the autumn trees that line the horizon and the fields before. As I returned I recalled the cornflower here, now gone, whose image lit up my retina and will live on in my mind for as long as my neurones fire. I gravitated towards a pub, stopping off to investigate a gap in the hedgerow. I found a new wood to search. It was full of birdsong, hawk and buzzard.

A couple of days on, and the wind stirred the warm air through the trees, bending them from their base, the motion magnified as the branches thinned to branches, which were dragged further still by their crisp leaves. Between gusts the tree would rock back. As I walked leaves scampered the surface, jumping to greet me. It was a sky-darkening, roaring wind, the sonic boom of the afterburn of days before. The wind was urgent, stealing the blue, hiding the setting sun, but hardly cooling the air as it turned the screw and tested the resolve of the trees. Where blue remained, evidence of the sun could be seen in yellow-tinted cloud, but birds had abandoned the sky; the robin didn't care to sing.

The lake in the hollows vibrated and ripples chased the light. The floor of the wood was calm and leaves lay still as, above, the canopy swayed. The meadow to rookery wood had been cut once more and all was silent, apart from the wind. The trees had a blackness of green behind a veil of grey defeat. There was a haze of rain, but no rain. I joined the three oaks in the open meadow as the sky produced a hint of Mars. Turning to face the wind and look out over the field I was struck by the thickness of the air, the darkness of rookery wood against the grey, but the only thunder was the trailers of harvest rushing along the lane in the fading light. The warmth of summer was slowly deserting through a hole in space and time where blackness engulfed. It grasped the landscape through the air and had to be dragged from October where it dared to tread.

And then, a few days later, summer finally collapsed. The oxbow was as black as the crow, reflecting the remnants of the sun. Launched into cold, I scuttled the fields under liquid grey skies; forced into the dusk there was enough light to visit the painter's alder. I now perceived it as dark and collapsing, rather than reaching, for who would reach for cold darkness? Perhaps the snag tree, but not the alder. I flushed two mallards, their exit ringing the water before it returned to blackness. The cold wind ached my teeth, the rain came and I was on a grit-stone edge, on the moor, exposed, with my mac rippling with the drops.

Two days further on, it was twenty degrees cooler than it had been a week before, and ordinary things were as they should be. Finally my mind and season met under grey clouds at Dunstall. I saw autumn, I felt autumn and heard the autumn winds and that was where I was ready to be, with the leaves joining me on the earth, smothering the grass and filling the sky. I had been waiting since the golden birch of Northumberland in August to slip into the cool closure of the fall. The low grey clouds teased apart to reveal higher grey. A patch lit silver revealed the location of the hidden sun, which blackened the paired rooks which were busy above the meadow. The mighty beech transfixed the field below as I sheltered along the bridleway. As the hedgerows thinned, the wind tried to be my friend, but only stole my warmth as it stole the golden leaves of the hawthorn too. The berries sat tight and dark, too smooth for the cold grasping hand reaching through the foliage. The mighty beech called and I picked my way through leaning nettles and dried briers, across leaf-pressed mire to be at its base. I shared the view down across the field, the bridleway cutting across. I witnessed the theft of leaves that the beech had called me to see. The escaped and fallen rolled in the meadow and skipped into lifting spirals as the wind chased them down. Wasps hovered amongst the young pine as I left the beech past the plantation to lookout over the wider landscape and the context of the Trent Valley and Needwood risings. As my year-long search comes to a close, the bare landscape will be revealed once more. Many of the younger ash were as they had been, bare, with matt black buds already sitting in quarters, the waved lichens tight and bright on the twigs beneath. Whole sections of the plantation were now bare, offering little cover and a line of sight to the mature, still green, wood behind. The young and weak had succumbed to autumns winds. Yet it was the woodland floor that was covered in tanned beech, yellowing leaves of ash and stepping-stones of green sycamore; either dark or light, dependent on how they had landed. And then the murderous call of the hawk switched on my senses and I was alive to the life in the trees. A curdling cry followed, before a distant robin sought to return the calm. I set off towards its song and paused by the window in the wood where more birds sang of spring. I looked out and received the valley, the rising land towards me, the birds and the sky. I received them as a whole, and connected as a whole, as the oak receives, connects and gives as a whole.

The next day we took our normal route around Brankley, with Isla ahead, as we neared the corner to the leaning oak. Returning she said, "I've found a short cut. Can we investigate?" Through a gap in the shrubbery we did so, emerging into a clearing centred by another ancient oak, surrounded by shed branches and birch. Fallen leaves rested on a spongy leaf mould. It was a special place, a hidden space. This oak was more upright than its leaning neighbour, with one main spiralling upright, splitting and rejoining to support a substantial canopy. "I'm going to call it Isla's tree," said Isla, and it forever will be, in our minds at least. It is good to have a tree. The children attempted to catch falling leaves and then, in the mood to explore, Isla set off once more. Mission accomplished, she took me further, through laid holly with vertical shoots, caging the clearing. "Can we come in the snow? The secret place will be nice then," Isla asked. We returned to our planned route and approaching the leaning oak Isla spread her arms out: "the real old tree!" she exclaimed. We went to sit in the wood pasture looking out over the valley. Leon and Isla stood amongst a storm of leaves across the hillside and then, standing on the bench, shirt held out, Isla said, "I'm going to fly with the birds in the sky," before jumping and racing down the slope. Completing our circuit, shards of summer memories fluttered amongst the wizened plants. A ragged and faded brown argus butterfly rested on the purple knapweed and the last cornflower in the field margins, blue amongst the greens and golds.

There had been unseen night-time rain, soaking the darkness, and that evening I visited the swollen Dove. It flowed through banks of tired willow, past islands of green. The air was full and flowing too, filling my lungs and working with the sun to smear silver patterns on the river.

That night, whilst asleep, my mind took me to the landscapes I had seen in my father's slides. Scottish hills superimposed with a golden eagle that panned across, left to right. Photographs, the scenes others wanted to take away, the ordinary things they chose to capture when they pressed the shutter. I looked through the hundreds of slides with a new perspective. Summit panoramas, ridge ascents and clear sky views from brilliant snowfields above the clouds. The rising sun reddening the Matterhorn tip. The climbing routes off Llanberis Pass, Skye, and a chaffinch. All I have now is a photo voice and the cues of the landscape.

The scent of wood smoke touched the still air in the hollows as a moorhen stepped in half-flight, bringing light across the silted pool. The sun had set and taking time to see it would end in darkness, so I brushed my way through the curled crisp chestnut leaves. Humankind was being squeezed into ever narrower days, and paths crossed to the red half-light of rookery wood. There the robin sang, but the blackbird was only alarmed, having not sung since June. The autumnal evening tone to the light was somewhat otherworldly, a science fiction that wrote itself into another planetary sky to where a great horizon moon sat. The light lifted the green and reddened the earth as, at risk of being caught in the darkness, I took time to see. Returning, the drab pools gladly took the sky and from within the darkness of the hollows the landscape was as deep as it was high.

Laser-lit jewelled water cut the steel mist and sparked the leaves at Blithfield. The perfectly cool air welded to my skin as we moved amongst the ferns, which were freshly illuminated green to yellow with non-translucent golds. Through the dry air and forest floor to the dewy flower meadow, they returned to green with occasional ox-eye daisies making an October return. The blackberries in the hedgerow were wizened and black and the fallen, lichened branch still lay at the entrance to the wood, as it had all year. Here the fallen leaves were now fading, crisp and massed. A blackbird shot past the oiled snag tree pond and the alloyed mist about the bulrushes was woven by the birdsong of the unlikely dunnock. Broken fences were returning to organic, unstructured forms, and the beech rattled, its crisp leaves visibly vibrating against each other, flashing in the light and generating a static electric rainstorm, blown heavier on the wind and ebbing away as each tree was passed.

The next day the blanched grasses of Pool Green Wood were bright and dotted with fading bursts of tree foliage.

Beyond there were misted views to Callingwood and Needwood. I had come to a high spot to reacquaint myself with the tiring landscape. By the pools there was the brightness of a robin's song from within the crabapple. A pair of dunnocks called above the bulrushes. There was a peaceful, melancholy mood as the skylark took the distress of the jay away. Through the dense pine plantation, with layers of captured needles held aloft on either side, we returned through the calm. "I've just seen the fox, there in the bushes," said Leon.

Later, at Anslow the low sun revealed gossamer threads across the grasses, the light creating the base of a circle, a bright wireframe channel past the runted pool. A fox exited as I reached the top. I was too short for the lowering sun and rising beam that lit the cooling towers and would be flooding the plain by the Dove. It lit the salient ash, but this tree has not captured my mind. Nor has the corner oak opposite. I sat on the stile looking west, wondering what it takes for a tree to engage the mind and impress greater meaning on it. As I turned away from the sun, the clouds lay grey, like fallen stones, fired bright where the sun trailed. It emerged briefly to prick out a constellation on my retina that I could place anywhere in the sky.

I swept through the late landscape in a rush, with black trees against night cloud, faintly lit from technologies glow or a hidden moon. A sea of sound carried me over dark ground as storm air rustled, alive and tectonic beneath the comfort of the heavy cloud.

The sun's waning effect was symbolised by a frosted setting, and dusted pink clouds iced the sky beyond my slender tree and were mirrored to the east. The scene was set for frost and the cool air already engaged my exposed skin. There had been a rapid descent from summer-like highs, and the green hawthorn leaves hung limp. The crisp and sweet air was ready to deposit itself and coat the landscape in ever-increasing extremes. I was layered against the cold, adapting, but some things do not change. Always the shy heron and constant swan on the oxbow, as I passed the lifting moorhen and gurgle of the crow. I rounded the water to sit on the stump of a felled willow. The birdsong was plentiful, but as gentle as the sun's warmth. Birdsong is as gentle as air, for sound is air, it is atmosphere. Long-tailed tits joined me and I could hear their wings working the air as they passed to the hawthorn. A blue tit was amongst it, its primaries backlit as it progressed. Dragonflies clipped and quartered about the reeds as the quarter peal of the bells rolled across the plain. With the reflective water and taut air, the restful sounds surrounded. This was a real place that might be imagined, conjured and deployed. The blackbird was real, but refused to add its song, saving it for the coming of another ordinary year, when I will return too, for I have never seen this place in spring. A green woodpecker undulated bright over the flatness of the fresh newly sown green, before the clouds interrupted and the wind was unleashed and stole away the warmth, encouraging me to leave.

I continued to let the scenes from the height of fall flow through me, dousing the transistor switching of my mind, allowing my thoughts to flow like a mountain stream, channelled, yet free. I am flesh, not computer. That is why I need the woods. I arrived at Dunstall where cloud-free sky allowed the sun to pick out the snag trees in the berry laden hedgerow. The mited horse chestnut was almost bare, twigs looping earthwards before arcing up towards the sky, its lower branches hanging on to the limp hands of leaves, helpless, not even attempting to grasp the lively air that ran between them. Several trees still held a firm green, but most were turning, including the oak, which released its leaves to fly by me. Here too the green woodpecker was out in the open, teasing the yellowing trees. Through the window in the wood I flushed a dozen pheasants, which lifted in series, beating and choking frantically as they dispersed in various directions. It was visually autumn in the established woods, but there had been no rain to release the scent that connects the season completely. The ground was as dry as the leaves. Then, I tracked a large grey bird through the trees, taking the path of the hawk we'd seen in spring; it was probably a buzzard, but the new pigeon kill in the field beyond made me wonder if the goshawk had returned.

Of course, the prospect drew me back and the sky launched me away from the Earth to the depths of Europa where I looked up at the icy surface above and the sun's faint glow. Despite the icy sphere above, the air was warm and I went in search of the return of the hawk. Within seconds, from a couple of hundred yards away, I saw a second burst of feathers in the open field, a pattern not seen since the spring. I stood beneath the mighty beech, its leaves also turning, wishing my sight could penetrate the copse and give witness. There was plenty of pigeon traffic and I was fired on by bursts of colour in the plantation towards the thawing sun trapped behind fluid high cloud. Long-tailed tits barrelled around me, their chirps burrowing into my inner ear. Crows spread their wings, vainly attempting to cover the expanse of sky. A thoroughfare of pigeons raced towards the killing field and a green woodpecker emerged to tease the fading trees once more. I took time to watch and hope, but left as the sun cast me across the fields.

A few days later I chased the liquid sun down to Brankley, where low and sharp it jousted me into retreat across the fields. Dismounted, I stood alone within a 360-degree turmoil of cloud, exploding the horizon as if I were a meteor at the centre of a giant crater, amidst the falling debris of oak leaves.

And that explosion broke the dam that had kept the ground dry for so long. Rain came, accompanied by a grey filter that filled the day as autumn descended. The dank grey air somehow drew out the colours even though they were subdued. The cloud sat long and low, narrowing the landscape beneath a concrete slab. The fields tiled away, edged and dotted by darkness, until a dead end of horizon trees edged the sky.

The death of leaves had bled into the day and it was still. Single leaves stuck motionless to forlorn twigs, the burst of summer hedgerow growth frozen. And all the time the landscape received the rain, hour after hour. And, like a needle finding a groove, I was channelled to the hollows to witness the final washing away of the residue of summer. There was a frantic stillness in the air of the wood, with the stream, triggered leaves and ringed pools the only motion. With the sound there was an intense essence of the season. It was the beating, flowing, heart of nature. I soaked it up and changed state like the dry ground around me as the light faded to robin and further rain. Reflections, smeared by a retreating hand, hung below the static trees and across the lake the willow island was a joy of murkiness. Like a faded and blurred colour print from childhood enlarged to vast size, it had a captivating drabness. I consumed it slowly and left, drenched by summer and soaked by autumn, with the pulsating wood of dusk and rain behind me.

The sun rose and thick white mist layered the morning landscape, eventually leaving moisture-filled bright air. The oxbow was more reflective and all was golden where I'd sat days before. The willow, the hawthorn and the reeds eked out the best of the light, but the painter's alder was resistant, dark green, its reflection black against the dusk. Its angular trunk and branches were bright and defined by shadow. Different birds were busy in the aviary of birch. I ached at the glory of the sky reflected, starred by lone clumps of reed. The blade of autumn was cutting deep and I would soon be denied the dusk too. The crow showed its greater darkness and a heron, with crooked neck, left silhouetted against orange cloud.

139

Greylag geese stepped the grassland in sync, orange beaks bright. Gulls floated on the lake, white, and even the jackdaws were bright as they picked between the leaves beneath the oaks, their calls as crisp as the light. Each billowing sprig of oak leaf could be seen in distant detail, a fluid mass in the breeze. It was a wonderful sight to have on the retina and painted in the mind, all-encompassing, clearly well for my being, instinctively right.

At Dunstall mushrooms sat like pebbles washed from some far shore, but there was no sign of the hawk. I felt there was to be no reprise of April and a sense of a closing. Then the sun came from behind the limes to point out the beauty. Light rushed across the landscape, a solar storm to fire the top plantation bold against the grey cloud beyond. Colours were exposed like minerals of precious brilliance mined from the Earth, reflecting light as if for the first time: simple things as special as the errant hawk. The buzzard appeared, spanning the sky, lifting on the air to look down on the opportunities surfacing below. I'd clocked October and was moving on, wise to the landscape.

During the night the rain ebbed and fell, sounding out its rhythms and bending the leaves unseen. By morning the skies had largely cleared, just thin layers of thin cloud with grey stains racing across, like floaters in an eye. Trees, haunted by pumpkin hues, sat calmly, for it was now November and by the new noon the grey was complete and the rain had returned. I set out to explore the new colours and structures revealed at Dunstall, and the rain explored with me, touching every surface and pooling each hollow, but it was not without light. Branches darkened by the rain shone from their uppers, like lines of ice defining the fractal path of the edges. Pheasants left the fields on wing and foot, as the trees behind were masked. But not the mighty beech, deep in colour, its dark inner structure revealed. The rain stopped and I watched sprigs of ash leaves glide in stable spirals to join their kin spread amongst the grass below, whilst a blue tit ratcheted its call behind me. The Earth tugged the water droplets from high in the trees and pigeons exited their failing cover.

The intensity of the colours had increased again, approaching their zenith, yet the silver poplar, hidden all summer, stood and eclipsed the brightness of them all. Once again I was forced to attend to the paths and my footwork, just as it was becoming possible for my vision to penetrate the trees. Blue and great tits were revealed in the plantation which topped the hill in stark contrast with the departing leaden cloud, but I soon re-found the rain as I found the buzzard's perch, a bare ash at a high point looking out over the Trent Valley. There was a light of midday dusk and a still acceptance of the season. The remaining leaves were individuals in their own space, each clearly the same, yet clearly different. Together, their hues changed the quality of the light. The asana trees were poised once more, but tipped by silvered browns. Equally poised was the clover, each leaf balanced a single droplet of water at its centre. Close by was a lone dandelion in late flower. In the darkness of the wood a streamlet carried the light and I followed to the open fields to accept and be contented by the heaviest ripping of horizontal rain. It stole the colour of all but the brightest and closest tree, and I was drenched.

Then came a vague, slippery day with little to take hold of and, desperate not to waste the shortening days, I set off on a slow exploration of the hollows to find something in the vague light and vague air, which was neither bright or dull, cold nor mild. Within the wood I stood and it came to me. The gentle motion of the lake gave impressions of the trees, not a mirror to the world. Each leaf was a brushstroke, crossed by the parallel compressions and expansions of the light, peeling the tops of the trees free, before returning them, and making the birds hop across the reflected sky. After reconnecting my vision, I stood and listened. I heard the passing stream and the distant jackdaws lifting around my slender tree, the silver sky beyond tinted by the weakening and falling sun. The stalks of the harvested maize amongst the sodden soil gave a foreground of devastation as they explored every angle and bearing from their pool intersected rows. Like Dunstall in May, my senses were overwhelmed by the connection. I set off to circuit the field, only to be snagged by a wild rose. I was forced to stop and discovered I was standing within a few yards of a powerful beech. Straight, it had no twisting of the trunk and rose to a great height. As I completed the circuit, the low sun broke through; too low to light the earth, it engaged with every beech, highlighting them, into bursts of colour appropriate to the night ahead.

I was conscious of the closing of my year in search of ordinary things. It was ending, just as much of nature was closing down for winter. I felt that I should stop my search and rest with nature, rather than continuing to engage it, but whenever I have thought nature had nothing to say, it has appeared, like the kingfisher, bright and demanding attention. So I was drawn to the hollows once more. The earth was taking back what it could. A repossession, clinging to mist over dew-heavy fields, dense and coated with sodden leaves, which made what they could of the fading light. I stood looking at the still lake reflecting the five o'clock sky when a ring of dark water appeared, central and expanding. Not to a vanishing point, but from a vanished point to an ever growing and fading circumference. I saw my year, a circumference of the sun, and realised nature can know no beginning or end; there is none in our orbit, only what we impose. The year will be and it is just that I had made a greater effort to enjoy the ride. I felt confident that my sample of one had confirmed how great nature can be: always ready to engage with our internal world. Ready to excite. Ready to calm. Always there, as long as we allow it space and time.

In the clear night sky the moon attracts our gaze and from my night on Earth I could see day, night and dusk on our moon, and day on Jupiter. An hour after it departed for its long winter's night, the sky still gave away where the sun had set and the moon gave its reflected day to the orchard, to the owl and the fox. It was time to start the closing.

XII

THE CLOSING

7 November to 31 December

The Dove flood plain appeared flatter in the cold grey of a claggy November day, flat enough to see the lines of hedgerows and bank-top trees fade progressively into the season. "They're still there!" exclaimed Leon, looking towards the small patch of cornflowers, which were still holding out and dancing about in the breeze. "I like this weather," he went on, and I do too, but why we couldn't explain.

The painter's alder was still green, but now touching the water after the recent rains. The Dove was brown, ridden by cream spots of foam that revealed hidden currents. Funnelling past the bend where a dead space lay, a twilight of river where trapped foam flowed back slowly to be drawn into the rapid current where it was teased apart to be reformed at the exit of the bend to drift slowly on once more. There was no light to play with the ripples; it was diffuse and intermingled with the moist air. Instead the sounds highlighted the location. On the bank, leaves from a single willow lay separate in the grass, only occasionally overlapping despite their number.

I returned to Anslow to find the pool still diminished despite recent rains. The trapped weather front had moved on and it was clearer. Structural trees stood subdued in the hedgerows, with a stillness of winter about them. Blackening vegetation was slumped between the plantation trees, many of which still had brightness attached. The birch were particularly fine, with their keen twigs and dotted splashes still picking out their wireframe form. The corner ash was bare, but not the corner oak, its diagonal partner. The open grey sky turned every bird to black, even the disparate dancing cloud of thirty finches, which crossed above the plantation with unseasonal glee. A small dew-laden web sat in the grasses, with dewdrop-formed sparkled circles creating a new butterfly's wing. Where I'd felt the breath of winter in January, the blackbird's alarm call had unusual warmth and, with a content freedom from purpose, I joyed the birch-created channel; my slender tree in the distance before me. I felt that I had found what I was looking for.

A few days later a mist of opportunity called me to Brankley. That visible, but intangible, state that engulfs all, human or nature, and connects it. Despite the sunshine of the day, the early morning mist had not fully cleared and by sundown its grip on the landscape was being re-established. But not so much so that the sun couldn't play a part, highlighting the subdued glory of autumnal oak, fading into the mist as they finally lost their green. The hedgerows were an illuminated frieze in bas relief, the tempered sun barred and released as I progressed to the final fluttering delight of the young birch. In the other place beyond the leaning oak, the grass was dense with moss and various fungal forms. Of all things, a pigeon feather captured my attention, its crisp border of white skirting a smooth greyness of blue, split by a rachis that blended from contrast through to unity of colour. A distant oak drew me away, its dead branches violently spiralling out from the explosion of colour where its bole divided. With a setting glow visible through the treetops and grey wisps of cloud above, the wood looked ablaze, and I retreated to await another day.

In that day, nine slender trees stood against the sun, only the uppermost branches retaining leaves, like flame-tipped rockets at re-entry. Next to them was a rounded form, revealed only by the backlit leaves through the light morning mists. A trio of black shadow-like arcs giving away its superstructure. Minded to explore less frequented haunts, the shoot had funnelled me back and forth across the landscape to return to the familiar paths at Dunstall. The hawthorn hedgerows were darkening; highlights dropped, berries deep, brightened only by hanging rain. Below was a cloven-petalled lone flower of red campion, topped by a curved flourish. Nearby, teasels were dark masses within the curving spent grasses, dense moments in space, brown dwarfs in a string theory.

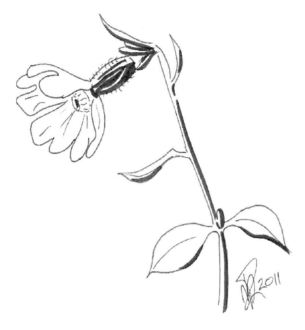

The lightly clouded sun was gentle, adding delicate relief to the fields, shadows not stark and grass, wet with overnight rain, subtly bright. The warmth and light breeze combined to create an autumnal rather than wintry scene. I sensed balance, and stopped to do less and notice more. I listened to the wood, watched the paths traced by the birds as oak leaves spiralled. A dead beech I'd not registered before, nuthatch climbing, detached branches hanging, a darkness of decay. A squirrel ran a fallen trunk, stopping to tend rapidly its silver-tipped fur. Lone ladybirds were snug, wagtails caught the sunlight as they had on the Dunstanburgh coast in August, and I felt the need to seek out the coast once more.

My travel complete, the sonic undercurrent of the sea was constant across the solid, open sands, as constant as the sun's flare reflected by the wetness. The sand was dressed with individual reflective points as the tops of the surf blew free, reminiscent of a snow-covered summit in the wind, a wind as firm as the water-patterned beach. The wind decorated the film of sea and blew sand to circle the moated rocks. The blown sands snaked the surface in inches-high storms and, like a satellite above the jet stream, I watched their progress as Isla placed her hands to be blasted by the grains. Nature was not in retreat here; it was gathering strength, its raw energy balancing the calm repossession inland. Here there were no trees in sight to give away the season, and I had a new perspective on autumn.

The unseen sea filled the night, the broad sound weighting every neurone and blanketing all thought. Morning light revealed the wide band of breaking waves weighting every grain of sand and blanketing the beach. The sea was extracted of colour to base grey. Every ocean point took its turn to rise and fall, to roll and break and to be blown to spray. Baggy Point sat in a darkness of spray underlined by broken white lines. Further west, Hartland Point was just a shade of grey away from the sky. A pied wagtail flicked its tail as waves piled the beach.

Further on, violent formations of rock ripped and spiked the breaking waters, angular as the thorned bushes before. Waves broke along their ripped apex, releasing trailing plumes, like feathered war bonnets charging the plain, to engage with the land in crazy chemical ferment. At Morte Point the bones of the landscape were revealed like the branches of an angular winter's tree, forever fractal with ever closer inspection. A challenging, rather than connective, landscape where the rawness of nature is exposed, befitting of the local saying, "Morte is the place which heaven made last and the devil will take first."

Back on the open sands gulls occupied the sea-filmed beach against a setting silver sun. Each expanse of calm between the waves was lit and stepping towards the horizon. The waves gave everything before fading to sheets that slid along the sand as the light also slid in obliquely. Repeatedly the gulls took flight on my approach, to land further on, stand reflected before stepping into the air, low, beating their wings as one. As we turned to walk with the wind the gulls lifted seawards to skirt us. A pair of sanderlings busily ran by the water's edge, at ease against the reflected blue.

The next day we walked a sunken lane to journey from country to coast and I found a single white rose high in the hedgerow. With its dusted yellow middle it dominated its tiny leaves, and the hedgerow. We left the lane through a tunnel of shrubbery towards Bennett's Mouth. Mosses and fresh grasses stark against the leaf mould gave this hidden valley a buzz of spring. At the base of our descent was a stream of perfect clarity and tone, finding its way amongst heavily lichened and mossed hawthorn trunks. The liquid sunshine washed the beech leaves and bounced off the ivy before flowing with the stream, bridged by long fallen trees, towards the sea. As the valley opened, grey trees stood against bronzed fern, as did highlights of yellow gorse amidst a mess of individual beauty. Shining as if alight, molten bronze berries dripped amongst the dried ferns, unlikely balloons above the thorns of the bramble. Where the stream met the sea I stood so that I could hear them both and feel the wind and the sun against my skin. The settled spray worked with the sun to highlight every edge of rock. Isla called me: "Daddy, come and sit here! It has a hand rest, back rest and food!", as she offered her sherbet pips. We sat facing the valley and the sun, with the sea behind us. "I love it here," she said, and this one half-mile valley alone could sustain me. From above, the valley was filled with a cushion of green, its snug position in the contours of the landscape revealed. I returned to base, sat in the warm sun above the sands, and consumed a Barn Owl, brewed to aid the conservation of owls for the Hawk and Owl Trust.

I then retraced yesterday's path along the coast. Seeing Isla's footprints made me wonder what trace she might leave on this world. It is a human thought, not one of wildlife, and I looked out at the trace of millions of years of nature, the geology exposed and life evolved, and felt that we should aim not to leave a physical trace on the Earth, just a positive trace in the mind of others. I soon left it as a conundrum that doesn't need my answer and decided to attend to the present: the light on the rocks of Morte Point, faces reflecting silver as they stood out, aggressive against the pinked drawn clouds. The three miles of surf snaking the bay, encompassed with ease by the sun's reach as its sharpening presence fell to set on my search of the coast.

Back home by the oxbow, the light and grey sky were as flat as the flood plain and a still mist faded all that was distant, giving an added perception of depth and calling me to dive in and explore. Even in the greyness, the clump of blue cornflowers remained to lift me. The silence carried the intermittent call of a crow, then of the fieldfares, the fluttering of a chaffinch and trill of a wren. The willows now just hazed the grey with a hint of past gold, their fallen leaves brown and returning to earth. Nearby the painter's alder was still stubbornly green, reflecting in its angle. Its reflection captured its form better than its reality, pure against the sky, every outline of its structure picked out in the calm darkness of the water. Closer, I found the alder was releasing some leaves and they lay dark on the bank around its trunk, a silver-grey of Morte Point rock. There was a glorious aching stillness of powerful affect, contrasting and surpassing the intense energy of the morning's coast. I was charged by the power of my familiar landscape and I felt alive in the stillness, as a star is bright in the night sky. Where the river was audibly unstill I looked out over the flat lands, from foreground to far, and felt that the landscape and my mind merged, my sense of self dissolved. I had arrived to dull shades of grey but heard the song of the Earth.

I returned to Dunstall, the field heavy with jackdaw and rook, but it did not speak to me like the Dove just days before. Baring trees were buffeted by the wind under a sliding sky, revealing the sun on occasion. I felt January's detail as the low sun challenged my eyes. I stopped in a plantation to give nature time and soon saw the differences in form of the bare young trees. The laddered cherry, gnarled ash and fresh year's growth of the lime, elegant curves with asymmetrical buds stepping to a paired tip. An ash weaving its near neighbour in tight embrace. White poplar leaves, like powered white prints across the earth. A single rose petal lay between, wet and cold, looking faded from pink rather than white-edged with warmth. Above was another fooled rose, teased by the mild weather, with fresh green growth amidst the hips imploding to darkness.

A couple of days later, walking towards the Tad Arm of Blithfield, varied fieldfare greys filled the sky on a day in between mild and cold, in between autumn and winter, in between the start and end of my search for ordinary things. A day when so much was ordinary. Ordinary turning leaves. Ordinary birdsong. But that is what made it so bright. I was surrounded by ordinary things, bird calls all around, the speck of a goldcrest, like a powered falling leaf. A treecreeper helter-skeltered a trunk, spiralling up, then down in the air, never more than two feet away from the bark. A tree stump with clustered masses of fungi over it, like waves breaking against a rock on the shore, building from the base to spill over the plateau. I climbed too, crashing through fallen leaves up a bank to be level with the canopy of marl-pitted sycamore, their yellowed leaves still broad, held in level balance to catch the summer's sun. Their slender trunks and branches strained to reach the level of surrounding trees.

I heard the wind working its way around them, the creak of swaying pine behind, and on occasion a single lobed leaf would spiral down to the ground, sometimes close enough to be heard if the wind had fallen to a lull of tranquillity. Then I realised here there was no birdsong. I walked for a few miles more, with clarity and joy, before being diverted as two hundred disturbed geese, in broken chaotic formation, squabbled the air space between the heavy-paned water and cloud.

Night passed and the sky-blue light shone the yellow oak leaves green as the wind dragged across the glistening landscape, accelerating the Earth and the fall. Hazel branches were silhouetted against a backdrop of remaining bright leaves, dynamic in the wind, tight catkins in trios and pairs. The crisp exact light brought the landscape to my eyes as the midday sun cast shadows long.

As the sun inched towards dusk I set out to where I knew the light would flood the oxbow plain. Tree shadows stretched a hundred yards and the golden light lifted the green, as opposed to last week's grey. The lone hedgerow oak glowed, complemented by the sun's late hue. The painter's alder had given its leaves and was now husked. Fieldfares lifted, like shining chaff from the red-starred hawthorn on the opposite bank, as the heron crossed the meadow in nap-of-the-earth flight as low as the sun's rays. As I returned, bank-top willow, birch and hawthorn strobed the horizon-sitting sun.

Chased clouds, lone and en masse, slid across the sky, lining up to bring darkness, or reveal the blue of the closing November sky. Dunstall was crossed by the wind. There was a deep roar from a tree resonant to the speed of the gale and bulleted larch peppered the plantations. I glimpsed the crescent of a low departing buzzard amongst the myriad airborne leaves that were mirrored by the rooks and jackdaws as they lifted as one from the field, like ashes drifting above a burning valley. My wider circumference of Dunstall under changing skies was a reprise of the year. I felt the entirety of my search and the completeness of the landscape. It was difficult to comprehend, and the clouds gathered into darkness, bringing rain and closing the daylight with a wonderfully bleak melancholy drabness. Rain passed, the dark sky cleared, cloud was rippled by the wind as the sea moulds the sand. Then, fronted by shots of low cloud, a tangible bank of earth touching darkness appeared to march before the horizon to reunite with the departed storm.

A totally blue December sky expanded over Brankley, allowing the sun to highlight the remaining autumn hues. The colours of the landscape were becoming subdued and the wind bent the scruffy grasses that were returning to winter beige. We were here to explore and a silvered rabbit tunnelled the hedgerow as we entered new pasture. Through clumps of grass, spines on the back of the living Earth, we reached a copse where the tree trunks were a tired olive beneath occasional coned pine, very much alive with green. It was sheltered from the wind and December's trace of warmth gave reason to pause. With time the colours of the tired copse became more vivid, red berries, bronzed ferns and hidden birch trunks slashing down. Turning to take in the commanding view to the south, a buzzard passed over to settle in the copse. "I like it up here. I like that tree," said Leon whilst looking at an aged oak, smattered by leaves and with a fallen branch at its base. Leon sat on the branch and I looked on as he watched the buzzard flow away. We crested the hill and explored Lockley Plantation where the course of the wind was decorated by crisp sounding leaves. We covered more new ground, pushing on through the wind until we were jolted as we escaped into the larch wood that swayed against the blue. Away from the paths, it was undisturbed, and skeletal bluebells still stood amongst sunlit ferns. We found our way back to a familiar route by the leaning oak and I ran my hand over the ancient holly trunk nearby. We sat in the landscape, opposite a compassionate oak and falling through the wind, as buzzards soared above. As we returned we stopped beneath an oak to watch the leaves fall against the blue. Each taking its own route, some spiralling slowly, sun lighting each aspect in turn, others frantic in their fall. Greenfinches passed like leaves returning to the trees. "I think I feel part of the landscape now," said Leon.

Later, I travelled the Trent Valley floor like a river, banked by sunshine and the risings beyond. Returning to the lagoons at Drakelow, the landscape cued my mind, and my trip was also all those that had gone before. Not stratified experiences trapped in the flesh of my mind, but an internal mind-wide web with distributed nodes in the landscape. The lagoon was a network of wildfowl, their wakes a matrix layer beneath the cormorants looping counter-clockwise into the wind to land on their snag perches, lit high by the floored sun. Against that sun the lagoon became a monochrome complexity of waves and crossing shrubbery. Opposite, a faded palette described the neighbouring pool and its blanched reeds. As the sun became a bearable disc, the light warmed and lifted the hue of the high branches and I made mindful progress towards the half-disc moon before it was lost to passing clouds.

I reached the point where time had passed whilst the dunnock sang, many months before. The breeze washed the reeds as the sea washes the shore. Back on the lagoon, the swans spilt their white and floated in its pool, as targeted coots contrasted nearby. Then a zephyr was mapped out in the water before it reached out to touch the reeds.

The next day brought a winter stillness; spent oak and birch sat contorted above the twisting stream further afield at Down Bank. Only the highest birch found movement in the air as gravity pulled the water through. It was weather for solace, so I headed for Brankley to explore its edges further, under increasingly heavy rain. A sparrowhawk passed by the steady kestrel and the bare trees were crisp despite the gloom. I skirted the newly discovered wood. Half-drenched trunks stood amid the bracken and yesterday's roar was replaced with sound of rainfall on autumn surfaces, which was both restful and fired the landscape. The green meadow opposite rolled to a crest that halved the line of trees beyond, their trunks hidden so that tips sat on the hilltop against the solid cloud. This new path took me to the place I wanted to be. An alarm call showed that the blackbird still had voice, but chose not to sing. On the corner of yesterday's copse a massive oak soaked up the remaining light in its stout trunk and thick branches. As I passed, its three-dimensional form was rotated and revealed, it seemed its energy and growth had gone into fewer corpulent divisions.

Clouds like frost blown across the sky were swept at length against the grey and the air was cold. As, to the north, a broad stunted rainbow became apparent, static against the cloud. Over several minutes it extended upwards, its arc seeming to be swept further by the winds until it reached its zenith and made a more rapid descent to the horizon to complete the arc. It then became faint and evaporated much more quickly than it had formed, to leave a standard winter's sky.

The strong low sun shining oblique amplified the pulse in my wrist, reminding me that I am nature and powered by the landscape and stars, reminding me how sitting indoors we have lost that connection, and I set out to Anslow Park in search of that visceral and reflective connection that has also powered me over the past months. The trees were stark in the light and nervous fieldfares scattered from the berried hedgerow. The pond was still just three large puddles in pitted mud, surrounded by oriflamme reeds in the gale, glowing gold and silver. Nearby, ash-tipped ash were lit to steel sculptures, each trunk, branch and twig lined by the light. Warmed by the sun I paused. Hoping to merge with the landscape, I focused on a compassionate oak and felt that I could see the wind. Then a buzzard graced before me to perch in the corner oak, before launching and leaving to become a notch middled arc.

At Brankley the next day, Isla smashed and skated the ice. Nature had given a new sensory experience to the landscape. "I like the ice. Feel it! It's really hard. I love cracking the ice," Isla went on, before we set off. Entering the field she continued, "I love frosty mud. Why does the mud get hard?" I felt the texture of the land on my feet, the bark on my hands and the cold air on my face. Isla said, "The fields are nice" and the sun had brought the greens to life and opened the wood that had been closed the week before. We identified the larch, pine, birch and "there's an eye", said Isla, pointing to a beech trunk. We circuited the wood so that the sun came through it to us, barred, lost and then apparent, whitening the bramble leaves beneath a bevy of bullfinches, their colours and lines as crisp as the day.

Later, by the Dove the cornflowers had been leached by the frost that had hardened the oxbow. The matt ice shattered in tracks, leaving panes of unnatural angles. The ice tempered the reflection of the painter's alder that was thick with cones. Shorn of leaves and navigated by chaffinches, it whispered, but I was in need of nature's voice. I walked on, diverting my course for the flow of the Dove, following a sense of where was best. The sky got broader and the land flatter, as my mind opened out from its closed focus. Whereas the oxbow was frozen, in water, in time and sound, here it was dynamic, the babbling Dove. Beyond the quarter-mile bridge I found an army of fieldfares, chattering like distant tanks rolling in to claim territory and occupy my thoughts. As the sun set behind a ridge and furrow sky, the ice of the oxbow chilled the air tight across my skin.

And then nature brought me rain and I returned through water-heavy lanes, flushing finches and fieldfares along the oxbow. The earth was as sodden and slippery as my connection to it beneath heavy skies. The tarnished painter's alder was free to touch its reflection, a reflection ringed by the drops from its origin. The Dove carried the rain away in a grim parade between hawthorn, ash, alder, oak and willow, all wearing black. The berries were the only evidence of the summer campaign, blood shots above a single white lens. From the edge of darkness I watched the Dove depart. A hawk left too, and across the gloom the distant trees raised from the flood plain to a height of grey mist. The advancing gloom lifted my spirits, as the landscape folded in around me and just the painter's alder remained bold. This was not like the joy the sun brings, but a contentment of solace.

Then came a cold, bright, but bland winter's day that wouldn't give me what I was looking for. I paced the fields and the exposed rookery wood felt hollow. I was thinking how nature cannot always bring relief. Then I realised I wasn't looking or making an effort, I wasn't keeping to my part of the deal to allow nature in. I gripped the tough cones of the alder and viewed the deserted beech, with few curled leaves remaining, nests revealed, branches laid down by the wind. An arched rose brier was hipped in the bleak hedgerow below. The pine still green above laddered trunk. Their shadows reached out across ploughed earth, dotted black and white with corvids and gulls. I felt relief well up. I left to follow my shadow across the clover until it was swallowed by the shadow of the oak.

At dawn I lay above the frozen earth, listening to winter's chorus, individual birdsong, the final drops of the year spilling into the cold air. The quad rasp of a crow, the punctuation at the end. Two-degree sleet on the wind arrived as if to test my desire to engage with nature; my end-of-year assessment. The sun shared my resolve and we set out across Dunstall, only for my companion to become little more than a flake of white in the solid grey as the snow in the rain

157

peppered my view. It was certainly immersive and the lid of cloud sat over Dunstall, brightness to all edges. The bicolour clasped shell of a nuthatch explored the base of a structured oak. My persistence through the conditions was rewarded when I reached higher ground. One hundred redpoll, or more, high in the birch, sounding like beads of glass on glass, hanging like baubles as I stalked through the young trees to get a closer view. On occasion they would launch as one, an explosive whoosh engulfing me, before they circled to return. The sky cleared to blue, reflecting my joy as the new light rested on the young ash, vertical and shining like precious metal spears in the earth.

A day later, at the oxbow, swan-tracked ice betrayed an earlier journey beside shadow-lined fields. After a freezing night with sleet, a rioting brightness from the released sun swept the plain. Our footsteps were crisp as we approached the painter's alder, half black by driven rain, and crossed by its own shadows. Beside the flowing Dove the water reacted angrily to the concrete weir in its path, clawing at its base, agitated from its gentle progress. Leon and I carried on upstream, crossing counties to be spooked by a low swan, its neck curving left and then right as it approached the field to feed with fourteen others. Our arrival caused three to pile into the air, one landing a hundred yards further away, the others circling before and above us a few times before departing north. We were surrounded by the veined winter forms of lime and maple, gathered in packs, circled by a buzzard. From within we stood and watched the bird life pass: moorhen, blue tits, robin and fieldfares, invisible until they took flight at our movement. Many left, but each step revealed more until we had passed and then returned, satisfied.

The shortest day arrived and the sun took hold in cloud-free skies and mild air. I was drawn to the leaning oak at Brankley. The young birch, which had been so jolly, had retreated into the blanched grasses, each holding a few memories of summer in their remaining curled leaves.

Clumped holly berries massed against the blue by the gateway to the wood, home of the leaning oak. In the pasture beyond, the noon equinox sun cast my shadow out across the landscape to point at an ancient oak. And there we stood, the circumference of our star nearly complete.

The payback for the brightness of the solstice was a day of rain. Continual, pulsing to a surface hazing onslaught, leaving a solid light filtering sky that tempered the next day too. Until it was cut open by a sparrowhawk, a tear that grew until the day was blue. The swollen Dove swept away what remained of autumn, churning, spinning, exploring and testing the banks. Like the oxbow, the sky was rippled by the wind. I searched for the space and time to stop, to reflect on over 220 walks in nature over a year. I felt that I was spiralling homeward from my continual search, when, for a moment I thought I heard a blackbird sing. A thrilling tone, like dripping sunshine, of the new year to come.

The sun soon revelled at the prospect of longer days, rising to light the clouds red. The chaotic cloud cleared to pampas and feathered flabella fanning the sky.

My year had been pretty much free of frost and certainly snow, and the sun was still not done with the Earth. It was mild and a little boggy as we circuited wider Brankley to the base of the corpulent oak. "I love logs," said Isla as she lay on top of a felled trunk. "I could go to sleep here," she continued, before exploring further. The sun fanned out over the wider landscape, making special all that it touched, such as the purple-black stems of the dog rose arching to bright yellow sprigs of leaves in fives, dominating the wizened hips. As the sun withdrew, the landscape sank into a grey cloaked inactivity below a reverie sky, which left me feeling detached from it all. When nature sleeps we must dream of spring.

A day progressed and by the canal it was warmer than the day in late March when the house martins saved our spring. Beneath the cabled sky a crow, beak glistening rook-like, swung in low over the pond to drink. Quenched, it rose four feet to perch on a post and release its corvid boast. The consecutive days seemed to merge under the glacial skies that crept over the landscape, swept by the finery of essential ash and lime. At the oxbow I was greeted by a kingfisher, an escaped plasma of all that is light, a point of intensity in the gloom as it floated past, silent, to perch. Yet even this could not ignite the awe of spring, the surrounding landscape being so subdued. With a connection to nature established I realised that I could not expect the excitement of spring from the recuperation of winter. Content with explanation, I walked calmly for some time, until the silence was shattered by the screech of the heron. I returned to the oxbow and tried the trick of sounding the call of the kingfisher. To my surprise, within seconds, the kingfisher flew past, wings pausing for a moment to glide yards from my feet, orange undersides a cross against the liquid coal below. It perched some distance away for a little while, before returning to the Dove.

The last day of my search for ordinary things in nature, as the year drew to a close. I had taken time to engage with nature, finding joy in my perception of the outside world as it had flowed into my mind. In the beginning I paid attention and slowly became more aware of the detail in my simple landscape. The ash was now my friend, when once I passed it with disregard. Each time nature spoke, I had to listen, and I found nature always had something to say. I had been attentive to the resulting thoughts and feelings, engaging the visceral, behavioural and reflective building blocks of my mind. I have experienced myself and the landscape differently and certainly had mindful moments, firmly in the now, but also pleasure in the unknown observations yet to come and the points in the landscape that prompt memories of my search.

During a year discovering how nature interacts with the mind, the landscape becomes an external memory, each haunt a scene full of cues. Many cues, like leaves on a tree. Locations and plants that trigger recollections from a year's search, the stile where the fox cubs played, the lagoon with an exhilaration of swifts or the post where the interstellar barn owl perched. Each path, plantation and tree, each flower, grass and bird, is connected to another time. Each scent and reflection, each cloud and gust of wind, both a present connection and memory weaving me into the landscape. The Needwood landscape means more to me than it did before, a hard-wired connection, and each landscape means different things to all of us.

Nature's cues also connect us with the past and future from our present, for we all see and hear the same things; as Waterton heard the rook, Baker the peregrine and Richard Jefferies saw it all. We can see the same, as our ancestors did, and our descendants will, but the effect of what we see depends on our mind. During my search I found a new way of looking at the familiar landscape. Just as flight can reveal imprints on the ground, when we travel to unusual heights of reflection our mind can penetrate the landscape and nature more deeply. This has led to feelings of excitement and release, but also the kindness of nature, as if it was aware and had complete understanding. Such as the compassionate oak, mature and safe; confident, supportive and accepting. I felt a very real connectedness to nature, a shift of awareness and emotion – completing a journey, although I've remained within a landscape. Just as I have found the comfort of my landscape, go and find the comfort of yours. Engage with it as you see fit, for there is no dogma in nature's glory.

On my final outing of the year, I set out to explore a new slice of the landscape, Crossplain Wood at Newchurch. Once again part of the ancient Forest of Needwood, but now a replanted narrow strip featuring an avenue of limes. Leon and I had visited before, but had been defeated by nettles. This time it was a day suitable to close a year; still, under solid skies giving drizzle. I passed a few pigeon kills before the likely culprit crossed my path: a sparrowhawk, which continued on, suitably silent, low through the plantation. Further on, rooks were about their nests, as jackdaws nearby popped and jibed. Below I found early, perhaps premature, signs of the new year to come, as fresh catkins hung still from the hazel. A magpie departed down the ride, an orb of white around its darkness. I continued along the straight, thin strip hearing only the occasional sound of the buzzard. I felt that I was walking through my mind, rather than the landscape. I slowed to a mindful pace, feeling each breath, and then a feeling beyond the limits of my language engulfed me and I wished that I could plant words as seeds. As the beat of the rain became apparent I reached a patch of old wood pasture where the most ancient oak seemed to reflect my condition, like a mirror of the mind. I stopped and I stood in the landscape, until only the landscape remained.

POSTSCRIPT

Having completed the writing of Needwood, I feel I need to acknowledge a couple of points. Firstly, the book does have an anthropocentric, or human-centred, perspective. At times, I do reveal a conservation ethic and the need to minimise the human impact on the Earth, but this was not the focus I set out with. However, as an emotional connection to nature predicts pro-environmental attitudes and behaviour I do believe that connecting to the local landscape is a simple first step towards more sustainable human behaviour and ethical responsibility towards the natural world. This is perhaps a situation where our own well-being might be a small step towards nature's well-being.

Secondly, and related to the first point, is that the introduction to Needwood represents a point in time where I considered the interaction between the internal mind and external world, but a connection to nature is more than a stimulus and response. It is more like gravity itself, a fundamental natural force possessed by all bodies, drawing them together, but waiting to be rediscovered. During my year-long search I gradually found this force and became more connected to nature, and the manifestation of this connection can be seen in this book. I increasingly saw myself as part of the natural world; I referred to the flesh of the Earth, flowed through nature's veins and felt the landscape and my mind merge – my sense of self dissolve. I started to realise that our flesh is inseparable from the flesh of the natural world; I had found deep nature. The natural world and landscape is not an external Other, something we encounter – it is part of our being. We exist as part of it physically and mentally. The depth of the landscape seemingly opens the dense flesh of the brain into space itself. We only understand the natural world because our minds are

163

embedded within it: we are nature's mind as much as our mind is nature.

Since completing my year-long search, I have felt compelled to look deeper into the thinking of others and have found that some have taken this path before me, such as the French philosopher Merleau-Ponty who equated the flesh of the body with the flesh of the Earth. I intend to journey further through the flesh of the Earth, considering embeddedness in the landscape along the way in a second book. Follow my progress and receive updates via:

www.needwood.net
www.facebook.com/needwood.book
twitter.com/richardsonmiles

PLAYLIST

Writing about our experience of nature requires reflection, which loses the immediacy of our primitive responses to the landscape. Music provides a further source of expression, and as a non-musician I have turned to the works of others which I feel help express my year-long search for ordinary things. To find the playlist visit www.needwood.net.

ACKNOWLEDGEMENTS

Special thanks to my wife Liz Richardson, for giving me the time and support needed to complete this work. To my children: Leon for his tranquil companionship; Isla for her enthusiastic insights, and both of them for their willingness to explore the landscape with me again and again. To Linda Allen, for chapter reviews and giving me the confidence to proceed. To the following friends, family and colleagues for their feedback on drafts, supportive listening and assistance: Richard Armer-Petrie, Ann Clark, Colin Clark, David Clark, Joanne Dalton, Jenny Hallam, Simon Lesley, Ian Mills, Glenda Richardson, David Sheffield and Perry Wardle. Jane Hammett for proof-reading. Finally, the custodians of the landscape and natural world around Needwood and beyond: Derbyshire Wildlife Trust, Staffordshire Wildlife Trust, The National Forest, Natural England, Woodland Trust, National Trust, Blithfield Estate, Rangemore Estate, Dunstall Estate, the Duchy of Lancaster's Needwood Estate and those others who maintain the various footpaths and rights of way.

BIBLIOGRAPHY

Sources of information and inspiration.

Allen, M. & Ellis, S.P. (2010). Nature Tales: Encounters with Britain's Wildlife. London: Elliott and Thompson.

Armstrong, E.A. (1940). Birds of the Grey Wind. London: Oxford University Press.

Baker, J.A. (1967). The Peregrine. London: Collins.

Brymer, E. et. al. (2010). The role of nature-based experiences in the development and maintenance of wellness. Asia-Pacific Journal of Health, Sport and Physical Education, 1(2), 21–27.

Clifton, S. & Windrum, A. (1997). Trent Valley and Rises. Natural England.

Coleridge, S.T. (1895). Anima poetae: from the unpublished note-books of Samuel Taylor Coleridge. London: Heinemann.

Emerson, R.W. (1836). Nature.

Ford, D. J. (1999). Land of the Dove. Leek: Churnet Valley Books.

Gilbert, P. (2009). The Compassionate Mind. London: Constable.

Griffin, A.H. (2005). A Lifetime of Mountains. London: Aurum Press.

Hartig, T. et. al. (2010). Health Benefits of Nature Experience: Psychological, Social and Cultural Processes. Chapter 5 in: Nilsson, K., et al. Forest, trees and human health. New York: Springer.

Howell, A.J. et. al. (2011). Nature Connectedness: Associations with well-being and mindfulness. Personality and Individual Differences, 51 (2), 166–171.

Jefferies, R. (1885). The Open Air. London: Chatto & Windus.

Laws, B. (2010). Collins Field Guide – Fields. London: HarperCollins.

Lister-Kaye, J. (2010). At the Water's Edge: A Personal Quest for Wildness. Edinburgh: Canongate.

Nisbet, E. et al. (2011). Happiness is in our Nature: Exploring Nature Relatedness as a Contributor to Subjective Well-Being. Journal of Happiness Studies 12(2), 303–322.

Norman, D.A. (2005). Emotional design: Why we love (or hate) everyday things. New York: Basic Books.

Olmsted, F. L. (1865). Yosemite and the Mariposa Grove: A Preliminary Report. Yosemite Association.

Richards, B. (2006). Small Adventures. Informally published.

Russell, J. (1974). Climb If You Will: A Commentary on Geoff Hayes and His Club, the Oread Mountaineering Club. EXPO 4974.

Shepherd, N. (2011). The Living Mountain. Edinburgh: Canongate Canons.

Taylor, T. (2010). The Artificial Ape: How Technology Changed the Course of Human Evolution. New York: Palgrave Macmillan.

Thomas, E. (1906). The South Country. New York: Dutton.

Thoreau, H. (1854). Walden or Life in the Woods. Boston: Ticknor and Fields.

Underhill, C.H. (1949). History of Tutbury and Rolleston. Burton-upon-Trent: Tresises.

Viscount Edward Grey of Fallodon. (1927). The Charm of Birds. London: Hodder and Stoughton.

171

Lightning Source UK Ltd.
Milton Keynes UK
UKOW050436040912

198445UK00001B/27/P